The Jossey-Bass Health Series brings together the most current information and ideas in health care from the leaders in the field. Titles from the Jossey-Bass Health Series include these essential health care resources:

Negotiating at
an Uneven Table

Phyllis Beck Kritek

Negotiating at an Uneven Table

Uneven Table

Developing Moral Courage in

Resolving Our Conflicts

SECOND EDITION

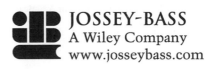

JOSSEY-BASS
A Wiley Company
www.josseybass.com

Published by Jossey-Bass
A Wiley Imprint
989 Market Street, San Francisco, CA 94103-1741   www.josseybass.com

Jossey-Bass books and products are available through most bookstores. To contact Jossey-Bass directly call our Customer Care Department within the U.S. at (800) 956-7739, outside the U.S. at (317) 572-3986 or fax (317) 572-4002.

Jossey-Bass also publishes its books in a variety of electronic formats. Some content that appears in print may not be available in electronic books.

Library of Congress Cataloging-in-Publication Data

Kritek, Phyllis Beck, 1943-
    Negotiating at an uneven table : developing moral courage in resolving our conflicts / Kritek, Phyllis Beck.— 2nd ed.
        p. ; cm.
    Includes bibliographical references and index.
    ISBN 0-7879-5937-5 (alk. paper)
        1. Negotiation. 2. Conflict management. 3. Nursing—Psychological aspects. [DNLM: 1. Ethics, Medical. 2. Conflict (Psychology). 3. Negotiating. 4. Nurse-Patient Relations. 5. Physician-Patient Relations. W 50 K924n 2002] I. Title.
    BF637.N4 K75 2002
    174'.2—dc21   2001006207

Printed in the United States of America
SECOND EDITION
PB Printing   10 9 8 7 6 5 4 3

Contents

Part Three: Constructive Ways of Being at an Uneven Table

This book was motivated by the children of planet Earth. Whenever I grew fainthearted, I thought of very real and particular children. These children helped keep me to the task:

Timothy; John Steven and Kevin; Maria; Tyler, Katie, and Emily; Tessa; Tim, Gillian, Mike, JJ and Erin; Daren; Josh, Tim, and Bill; Jeremy; Eric, Eric, Emily, and Emma; Peter and Jill; Gabe; Tracy and Toni; Bridget, Sheila, and Claire; Ryan and Nicole; Siobhan; Brett and Cary; Ryan; Katie and Amy; and Genevieve, Erica, and Jonathan.

This book is lovingly dedicated to the two children entrusted to my care: Patricia Anne Kritek and Rebecca Marie Kritek. It is their mother's hope that because of this book, they will know fewer uneven tables than she knew and will handle them with greater grace and wisdom than she did.

Preface to the First Edition

Negotiating at an Uneven Table is a book about negotiating conflicts in situations where some participants are at a disadvantage that others do not acknowledge. Such situations are considered uneven tables—places where the assurance of justice or fairness is uncertain or unlikely. When we are confronted with such situations, we hope that we can "even up" the table as a solution. Often we cannot. There are a range of possible responses to this situation. This book was written as a set of reflections on the options.

These reflections are personal and practical. They emerge from my life experiences and present my perspectives. More specifically, I have not set out to write a scholarly book in the traditional manner of the academy, but have intended rather to write an intelligent record of lessons from my life experiences at uneven tables.

Some of these life experiences have included training in and studying about conflict resolution. I have found these opportunities to learn and grow very enriching. I have also been haunted by the sense that something was missing, that my life experiences had taught me some things that were not explored in the studies, in the seminars, in the books, and in the courses on conflict resolution. This book is about what I think is missing.

My reflections therefore are not designed to provide a critical appraisal of conflict resolution, its theorists, practitioners, or scholars.

I am not attempting to unveil the deficiencies of others, particularly since I have such high regard for the professionals who are seeking to help us all resolve our conflicts more constructively. I do believe, however, that what I experience as missing can and perhaps will alter existing practices and approaches to conflict resolution. If this is constructive for others, that will please me.

It has been my experience that in the current climate in the United States, the response most accessible to the person invited to an uneven table is manipulation arising from an attitude of cynicism. This book posits an alternative. This alternative has asked more of me, but it also gives more back to everyone at the table. In the end, I believe it also serves to address conflict in a more creative manner.

My Aims, in Brief

I do not anticipate that in writing this book I will exhaust its theme, but I do intend to start a dialogue. I hope thereby to create new opportunities for dialogues about uneven tables. I trust and believe that these dialogues will go well beyond my insights, will further educate and enrich me, and will benefit others. I believe in the dialogue for its own sake.

I have experienced writing this book—my effort to start this dialogue—as a moral challenge. It is one I am not totally comfortable with, but one nonetheless that beckons, even compels me. The task is not pursued without trepidation. It has seemed to me that I have a very small margin for error. What can and perhaps should be said is often left unsaid, avoided, denied. I have tried to say some of these tough things in this book. Saying them well, in a "hearable" fashion, is also difficult.

It is my hope that my effort to write a careful and respectful book will enable others to respond. It is also my hope that those who find themselves at uneven tables will be encouraged to speak out on these issues. I further hope that you, the reader, will be better able to clarify your thinking about some often seemingly intangible but deeply troublesome human events and experiences that may have previously eluded your understanding. Perhaps this will widen the window on human possibility and lead to new vistas of creative responsiveness to human conflict.

A Brief Overview of the Terrain Ahead

In writing this book, I have tried to practice what I preach, to model the message of the book in how I have presented it. Because an uneven table is unveiled through an analysis of context, I have attended to context. Uneven tables tend to flourish because they are often unrecognized, so I have tried to provide you with tools for increasing your ability to recognize such tables.

Even if uneven tables are familiar, we often fail to explore new approaches to sitting at one. We have become habituated to traditional responses to an uneven table. I have thus described these traditional responses and demonstrated how they are usually deterrents to effective conflict resolution. The possibility of evolving beyond these traditional responses emerges naturally and leads to my description of ten "ways of being" at an uneven table. These ways of being have helped me to achieve constructive outcomes congruent with my reason for being at the table.

This brief overview presents an image more linear than either my thinking or the book actually manifests; both are more prone to matrix imaging. More simply, I believe any one part of the book can be read independently of other parts, but I know that what I am trying to communicate can best be understood as a part inextricably linked to the whole. Missing one part, one misses a significant dimension. Each part assumes that you have read the prior part, and all parts are related in an interactive sense of that term.

I have also included in this book some puzzle pieces, some reflections, and some exemplars. Sometimes I tell stories or parables and provide poetry or pictures. Occasionally I deliberately break the rules. Throughout the book, I suggest exercises you can do to test ideas and skills and to discover new things about yourself and others. I have tried to provide some moments of whimsy that might activate the child in you. I have done these things for several reasons.

One of the most challenging dimensions of negotiating at an uneven table is the need to know and acknowledge your own resistances and unconscious desires and goals, to unveil your own vested interest in warding off change. We can better experience such resistances if we are exposed to the same idea in two or more ways. Different modes of knowing provide multiple opportunities to discover personal blindnesses and vested interests, and make it harder and harder to keep the door closed to change. And change often requires that we break the rules.

We all like to think that we're pretty open-minded, which of course is true, unless we're asked to be open-minded about something where our minds are closed. That is why I have included in this book alternate ways of learning the same concept. This gives you the opportunity to activate multiple dimensions of what it means to be human, to tap into diverse ways of knowing and activating your multiple intelligences. It is my conviction that we will not become skillful at experiencing new ways of being unless we become comfortable at mastering new ways of knowing how to be.

This process need not, however, be all solemnity, pain, suffering, hardship, and struggle. The truth of things can be hard and demanding; it can also be funny and liberating. So, I've tried to introduce some fun to balance out the struggles you may experience as you go through the book.

Learning things can be difficult. Learning things that are painful or scary to face can be even more difficult. Some moments of self-honesty can be very challenging. A few light touches or funny exercises can help us stay at the tough task of becoming all we can become if we only have the honesty and courage to try.

It is my hope that all of this will make this book one of interest to you. I hope to start a dialogue and have sought to start the conversation as creatively as possible. You may actually find that as you go through the book, you will be inventing your own exercises, recalling your own parables, and remembering the stories that have shaped your experiences at uneven tables.

So, before you go any further, here's an exercise. Get a pencil and piece of paper. Now, flip back through this preface. Identify all the times that you wanted to say something back to me. Write it down. It doesn't have to be eloquent or clever. This is how a dialogue with a book begins. You may want to buy a notebook for this, since it won't be your last chance to write while you read. Take time-outs, enjoy discovery, reflect as needed. Dialogues are enriched by such decisions.

Acknowledgments

This book describes some lessons gleaned from living. I would like to acknowledge the two people who gave me the gift of this life, Paul C. Beck and Mildred A. Beck, and those who started the journey with me, my brothers, Bob, Leon, Paul, and Ken Beck, and my sisters, Rita Massart and Patty and Mary Beck. The other "big kids," Bob, Rita, and Leon, were directly involved in supporting me through this project, and as always, gave me the kind of consistent affirmation that has sustained me for years.

Two persons at Jossey-Bass played a central role in making this book happen. Trish O'Hare "found me" and my ideas and nurtured them to realization. Becky McGovern, my editor, did all the right things at all the right times and demonstrated a support and candor that I had not imagined possible. The fact that they have the same names as my daughters continues to evoke my reflective consideration. I consider each of them a special grace granted me, and am grateful for the gift.

The pragmatics of this task have unveiled my limitations, and several people stepped in to save me from myself. Irene Cvetich assisted in initial drafts of the manuscript, Mary Alice Hinch saw it through to completion, and Elaine Betterton chased down and ordered the references. Yvette Viator typed the bulk of the manuscript, with patience and enthusiasm. I am thankful for their contributions.

The Kellogg Foundation awarded me a National Leadership Fellowship in 1986, which gave me the opportunity to formally study conflict resolution and birth this project. The fellowship was for me the most valued educational experience of my career, and I thank those who made it such. Two members of my fellowship group, Lenny Marcus and Tim Dutton, played a unique role in that education, and I acknowledge my immeasurable gratitude for their support, challenges, and friendship.

I joined the faculty at the University of Texas Medical Branch at Galveston as this project was unfolding. Several colleagues there welcomed me into their community and served as a gracious support system: Bobbie Lee, Darlene Martin, Corrine Oppermann, Jerry Lester, and Martha Hargrave. Mary Fenton, dean of the School of Nursing, was consistently supportive. Phyllis Waters shared her rich energy and her spirit.

I have been blessed with many good friends who cheered me on through this process. Some contributed critical advice and comments, read drafts and revisions, or told me where I appeared to be going awry. Others provided a presence in my life that nourished me. Many did both. These people have my warm appreciation: Bill Bartholome, Nancy Beck, Warren Braden, Terry Brennan, Ken Cianfrani, Kris Gebbie, Eleanor Kirsch, Sara Looney, Shelly Malin, Jestene McCord, Bev McElmurry, Pat McManus, Pat Moccia, Carl Mueller, Greg Olson, Sue Pinkerton, Tim Size, and Linda Zwirlein. I am particularly indebted to two persons, Charles Gessert and Janet Krejci, who played uniquely catalytic roles in making this book happen, roles that defy description but not my deepest gratitude.

The most creative expression in my life has been my two daughters, Tricia Kritek and Becky Kritek. Their continued faith in me, their support, and their love sustain me in myriad ways. During the writing of this book, experiencing their sustenance was my refuge.

Finally, I want to thank the Gulf of Mexico for being and for being there for me.

Galveston, Texas   Phyllis Beck Kritek
August 1994

Preface to the Second Edition

I have taken the time to prepare this second edition a bit as a progress report. It is an update on what others—my students and the readers of the book—have taught me. I have also included the things I have learned from living in the light and shadow of this book for eight years. These insights are woven in along the way, sometimes in small ways and sometimes in big chunks.

I have found that I can affirm everything I said the first time, and want primarily to amplify and clarify some points. I am most interested in improving the scope or depth of presentation and do not offer any sudden shift in direction. Sometimes the ideas presented were not developed adequately, or with enough clarity. Where I could, I have attempted to correct this. What is stated in the Preface to the First Edition still holds.

One of the most interesting questions people have asked me about this book is, "Who wrote the poetry?" This always startles me a bit. To put the question to rest, and to lay claim to a dimension of my identity as a writer that I cherish: I wrote the poetry. It is another way of saying what I have to say.

There are some additional acknowledgments I wish to make in this edition. Many readers have given me helpful feedback through notes, e-mail, private conversations, and participation in workshops and training programs. They have shared what they found helpful and what they found unclear or confusing. I acknowledge all this help, which guided my work on this second edition. Some of these helpful ideas I now wish I had responded to more clearly at the time. As a first-time author, I was still in a learning mode. I anticipate that I will do better in the future. The many persons who have attended my workshops, lectures, and training programs on the content in this book have influenced my efforts in this second edition. I thank them for serving as both teachers and motivators.

Of particular importance to me is the group of students I call "mine" at this time because they were in the doctoral program I helped create and implement during the last several years. I want to thank them for their extensive feedback, advice, and constructive criticism. More than any other group, they were my teachers as I prepared this second edition. Some warrant special mention for their generosity, particularly Kimberly Crocker, David Crowther, Susan McConnell, and Ellarene Duis-Nittsche.

Jane and Reid Swanson have played so many supportive roles during this phase of my journey that I cannot describe them or my gratitude adequately. My secretary, Anita Padilla, has with great patience and kindness supported and guided me through the white water of my lifestyle. Carolyn Kinney, friend and colleague, has been both sounding board and spiritual force. Sara Looney, who kindles me with a friendship now almost forty years old, was a particularly critical force in moving me forward in this effort. I thank all these people for their gifts.

Sharon Atwell has played many roles beyond that of student in our shared journey. Her courage and wisdom, and the trust she inspires in others, are a beacon of light for me. Phyllis Waters is a soul connection that transcends the stories we tell. She is the strong healer in my life, and I thank her for this. Sue Pinkerton, Janet Krejci, and Shelly Malin have made friendship an art form in my life. They shared their ideas, challenges, and work worlds with me. I need to be near water to write; Sue provided writing retreats at her condo on the Atlantic, and Janet and Shelly did the same in their homes in Door County, Wisconsin. Hence, the second edition of this book was shaped by their friendships and the healing powers of the waters of the Gulf of Mexico, the Atlantic Ocean, and Lake Michigan. I am grateful.

Andy Pasternack was my editor at Jossey-Bass. He was the perfect person at the right time and has been responsive and supportive during this process; I thank him for being there and for his advocacy on my behalf. Perhaps most significant, he also let me be grumpy without recrimination.

Finally, although it is a given, I want to acknowledge my two daughters, Trish and Becky Kritek. I know that I did this already in the first Preface, and that this is repetitious, but during the intervening years our relationships have grown and matured in ways that have shaped this edition. Though they were entrusted to my care as infants, I find that as young adults they are my strongest support, my truest advocates, my best critics, and my protectors. I am in awe of their goodness of spirit, their courage, their creativity, and their capacity to love well. As before, Trish and Becky, this one's for you.

Galveston, Texas   Phyllis Beck Kritek
October 2001

The Author

Phyllis Beck Kritek is Florence Thelma Hall Distinguished Professor of Nursing at the University of Texas Medical Branch at Galveston School of Nursing. From 1993 to 2001, she served as development facilitator and director of a doctoral program focused on healing practices in nursing, editing a book on this theme. She previously held positions as director of the doctoral program in nursing and director of the Center for Nursing Research at the University of Wisconsin, Milwaukee, and as dean of Marquette University School of Nursing. She received her B.S. degree (1967) in nursing from Marillac College and her M.S. (1971) and Ph.D. (1980) degrees in nursing from the University of Illinois in Chicago.

Kritek is an internationally known nurse scholar. She has consulted or been a visiting scholar in Australia, Canada, Sweden, Brazil, Venezuela, Holland, and Mexico. Her interests have included areas such as nursing diagnosis, nursing research, doctoral education, organizational management, leadership development, mental health nursing, conflict resolution, gender issues, and the professional development of nurses. Her clinical practice is in psychiatric nursing, focused primarily on depressive disorders in women.

In 1986, she was awarded a three-year Kellogg Foundation Leadership Fellowship, which involved extensive national and international travel and collaboration with other Kellogg fellows on conflict resolution and gender relationships in health care. She has presented numerous workshops and training programs on negotiation skills, particularly for persons who frequently find themselves negotiating at uneven tables. She also provides mediation services for a variety of health care groups.

Negotiating at an Uneven Table

"Tell me of good and evil," I asked.
The old Indian replied,
"Inside of all people is
a good dog and an evil dog."
"Which one wins?" I asked.
He smiled a smile that only comes
with old age and wisdom, and said,
"The one you feed the most."
   —Story told by artist L. Don Mulkey, Galveston, Texas

Prologue

The evening of May 16, 1993, I was busy packing my luggage and savoring the anticipation of the trip I would take in the morning. I was headed to Boston to participate with a group of colleagues in conducting a one-week workshop on conflict resolution in health care. The colleagues were also valued friends, so I was looking forward to their companionship and stimulation. The workshop itself would be an exciting and creative one, and I was eager to begin the process.

Midweek, I would sign the contract for this book. My anticipation of this long-sought goal was intense, and I was pleasurably preoccupied. Some of the book's contents would be presented in the workshop the night before I signed the contract. I was imagining and enjoying the sequence of events.

The phone rang and changed both the fantasy and the course of events dramatically. My mother, eating out with one of my younger brothers and his wife, had had a heart attack at the restaurant and was in intensive care with a very poor prognosis. They had gone out to celebrate a belated Mother's Day and she abruptly slumped over. She was cardioverted twice in the restaurant and once in the emergency room. (Cardioversion is reactivation of heart contractions that stop, using an electrical current.) She was on a ventilator and was stable, but there was clear evidence that she had experienced prolonged oxygen deprivation. Her seven living children, one by one, were converging on the hospital.

My mother had left the same hospital only ten days earlier, after a frightening episode of pneumonia and the first signs of significant heart damage. She had been ill enough during this episode to have "lost" portions of the hospitalization experience and had been sobered by this new threat to her health. A lifelong asthmatic, she had decided fifteen years earlier between two options: a shorter but higher-quality life owing to use of cortisone in treating her asthma or a longer, lower-quality life without the cortisone. It had been a finely tuned process of medication management ever since.

After her discharge from this first hospitalization, she had moved expeditiously to contact each of her seven children and advise them of her current thoughts about her health status. She was a strong-willed woman, and her message was neither equivocal nor unclear. Some time earlier she had procured the information needed to file a living will. She had failed to complete the process but called each of us to make it abundantly clear that she intended to do so immediately. Indeed, the weekend of Mother's Day had been filled with phone calls and conversations with each of us, explaining the strength of her convictions. She did not want extraordinary measures, and she did not want anyone to misunderstand her intent.

Because my older sister and I are nurses, our conversations with our mother may have focused on the actual health issues in more detail. She assured us, as she had assured others, that she planned on seeing her physician the Tuesday after Mother's Day, and that she would explain all of this to him at length. She realized that it would take some time to complete the process, but she wanted him to know her decision now. They had known one another for many years, and she trusted him explicitly. He was the physician who had monitored her challenging health care over the years since her choice of a shortened but better life.

As was her style, she reentered her busy life following that hospitalization with a frenzy, determined to squeeze pleasure out of the life that remained. She enjoyed not only the Mother's Day celebration but also bridge and shopping with friends, altering clothing for the people who lived in her condominium, and following the diverse achievements of her children and grandchildren. Now, four days after telling her physician that she did not want extraordinary measures taken, she was in a hospital intensive care unit, breathing with a ventilator, hooked up to a monitor revealing the serious dysfunction of her heart contractions, and unresponsive to any external stimuli.

I canceled one trip and embarked on another, arriving early Sunday. Instead of teaching others about conflict resolution in health care or signing a book contract about negotiating at an uneven table, I lived both for three intense days, culminating in her peaceful death on the morning of May 19, 1993. It was a death as she would have wanted it, but one that we, her children, had to reclaim for her on her behalf. The journey was interrupted twice in the restaurant and once in the emergency room, and had we not intervened it might have been interrupted even more often or more dramatically.

In the book you now hold, I had planned to tell some of the stories that demonstrate the strange status of most nurses in our health care delivery system. Nurses are repeatedly asked to negotiate at an uneven table. I found such nurses in this hospital, and with my brothers and sisters I learned once more how well they do just that on behalf of patients and their families. The ones we worked with were superb, and they made the journey with us.

When I arrived, it became clear that those of her children who knew and understood health care would negotiate the relationships with the people in the hospital. I began collecting information, as a sense of foreboding grew in me. My younger brother knew that Mom had been without oxygen, had changed color, and had not responded to cardioversion with stability. Shaken and having already "experienced her death," he was haunted by the conversation about living wills in a unique way as he watched her breathe with the ventilator and watched the erratic patterns of her heart on the monitor. He and his wife had managed a terrifying situation superbly, but it had ended up exactly where she had told us all she did not want to be, ever.

I sought information from the nurses. They explained to me that they had been directed to cardiovert her again if needed. I asked why. They noted the physician had not given them a do-not-resuscitate order. I asked them if any kind of neurological appraisal had been made to determine how much brain function Mom still had. They noted that it was Sunday and that the necessary procedure would not occur on a weekend; it had been ordered for Monday. Meanwhile, they were continuing all of her medications, including her cortisone.

I asked if I could speak to her physician, and they contacted him by phone. I explained who I was and told him I was seeking additional information. He noted that Mom had been cardioverted three times and had never fully stabilized. He acknowledged that he knew she had been without oxygen for a long period of time, though no one knew how long. He knew that the heart damage was substantial— that she had been on cortisone long enough that the inevitable damages of the medication were now taking effect. He also knew that she was impervious to all stimuli. And of course, he knew she was a severe asthmatic, with all of the respiratory implications of that difficult disease.

I asked him why he wanted her to endure yet another cardioversion. He responded that he wanted "forty-eight hours" to evaluate the situation. I referred to her conversations with each of us about a living will, and he confirmed that she had discussed it with him also. He said he had told her he would want forty-eight hours. I told him that all of her children were worried about the degree to which we were showing a fidelity to her wishes. He became irritated with me and asked, "What are all these questions about, anyway? I explained all this to the family last night!" I noted that he had only talked with one of her children, the one who had stood by her through the disastrous night of events, who was not a health care provider, who was shaken and fatigued and stressed by the events he had witnessed. We ended the conversation somewhat tensely.

Having "hit a wall," I turned to the nurses in the intensive care unit for assistance and information. I explained that I was a nurse, and I slowly worked at gaining their confidence so they might tell me the things that I knew they knew but often were impeded from sharing. One of the cardinal rules nurses must always confront is the fact that if they differ with a physician, and the family and patient trust the physician, to create conflict can jeopardize the patient. Thus they must negotiate carefully and with great circumspection. These nurses knew all of this and were both respectful and careful with us. They would slip into Mom's room, attend to her physical needs, talk to her despite her lack of responsiveness, and all the while, I realized, listen to the conversations among her children to ascertain our status. They were expert nurses, and without really meeting any of us they quickly assessed the processes we were experiencing and sharing.

Slowly, it became clear to me that they too were troubled that they might have to once more cardiovert Mom. Even more gradually, I learned that they had been apprised by her physician on admission, "She talked to me about a living will this week, but we're going to treat her aggressively for forty-eight hours." The nurses, I discovered, were struggling with their sense of being coopted into doing something they believed was contrary to the patient's wishes. With the arrival of her seven children—none of whom are small or shy—they were absorbing an ever-more-intense level of concern about the strange turns her journey toward death was taking. One of my brothers stated in our discussions that maybe we would need to try to stop them if they tried once more to put her through a cardioversion procedure. Although the process might prolong her heartbeat, there was little evidence of a future state of recovery, and everyone knew that.

We became frustrated realizing that Mom might have to go through one or more cardioversions—partly because of the absence of a neurological appraisal of her status. Had the incident happened the night before a weekday, she would have had the neurological appraisal the next day. Had there been concern about the status of her and her children, there might have been an early reading of that appraisal and decisions about her status made that would have shortened the time she spent struggling to be released. Instead, we waited out Sunday, supported and sustained by a group of humane nurses and by one another. On Monday, they came early and did the neurological test that would tell us her status.

Optimistically, we looked forward to the information that would now be ours, knowing also that the forty-eight-hour plan was still in effect but hoping for early clarification. We waited all day, looking forward to information that might help us understand what we were collectively experiencing. We attempted numerous times to contact both physicians, and received no response. Prodding and prying with the nurses, we were advised that the neurologist had indicated that since he had not "come onto the case" until Monday, he too might need forty-eight hours to observe the patient. I requested a family meeting with both physicians so we might all tell the physicians what our understanding of our mother's wishes was, and to ask them how they intended to respond to these wishes.

I began to realize that although I was negotiating as best I could, I needed help. I called a physician ethicist friend who had extensive experience with these processes and sought his advice. He was exactly the supportive resource I needed, and slowly, step by step, he walked me through the things that we as a family needed to do. He presented the image that we needed to sustain us, explaining that Mom was caught between two places: life and death. If she could not realistically return through the door she had walked through, then she was in a corridor trying to get through some other door. We needed to make sure that all remaining doors were kept open until we could determine the viability of opening ones that had already been closed. With that image to guide us, we attempted to clarify our common commitment to giving Mom the kind of journey toward death she had wanted.

Meanwhile, Mom's death experience continued, and I watched Jill, her sixteen-year-old granddaughter and my godchild, struggle watching her struggle. Jill and Mom had a special connection, and

Jill knew her in a way most of us never would or could, in that way young persons can mysteriously connect with an old person who is also their grandparent. The ventilator forced a pattern of breathing unfamiliar to us all, since we knew her asthma well. The artificiality of the monitor, the sounds—all were dissonant with the woman who wanted none of it. "She would not want it this way," Jill whispered, fighting to make sense of the trap created for this woman who hated to lose control. My oldest brother, who is a priest, administered the last rites to her, and we prayed together, sang the Our Father that he had written and that she loved so much. The nurses guarded our privacy and our time, accepted and respected our prayer and song, and quietly assured us of their support. I knew again the awe I feel for the extraordinary power of good nurses doing good nursing.

I realized that if I demanded information from the nurses, demanded that they contact the physicians, they would of course then have to respond. They had limited power to act without our insistence, which gave them the reason they needed to provide us with information. I asked for information on the neurological test, asked what was recorded in the chart, asked which medications Mom was receiving, asked what type of nourishment she was getting from the IV and how much, asked what amount of oxygen she was receiving. From this information, I began to discover how much heart damage she had actually sustained, that indeed she still did not have a stable heartbeat, that she had evidence of minimal brain-stem function—perhaps enough to sustain a comatose resilient body for some time but unlikely to sustain a seventy-seven-year-old body without life support systems, and unable to sustain life. Clearly, the brain damage was massive, and we could anticipate no return to consciousness. At most, we might witness some erratic physical jerk or reaction, although we had seen none since Saturday.

Midday on Monday, after the last rites, the physician ordered that the nurses should try to briefly discontinue the ventilator to determine Mom's capacity to breathe without it. By then I was convinced that she would not be able to do so without the ventilator, especially knowing how hard she fought to breathe under normal conditions as an asthmatic. Had she never been placed on a ventilator, this process would not have been necessary. For a few moments, she appeared to continue the forced rhythm of the ventilator, then abruptly began to gasp for breath and go into spasms, and they had to reconnect the ventilator. My brother and his wife, already too burdened by the shock of their Saturday night experiences, left the room devastated, and we agreed as a family that they needed the freedom to not be there again for any procedure of this nature. As my brother said, "I've already watched her die once, and I can't keep going through this over and over." We all knew she was trapped then, and that the ventilator was necessary for her to be "defined" as alive.

As the time for the meeting with the physicians approached, we laid claim to a conference room and squeezed her seven children, three wives of my brothers, one grandchild, and my father—her former husband—into one little room. We made a space at the end of the room and placed two chairs for the two physicians. The nurses kept us apprised of the delays that led to their late arrival. They had conferred before they came in. The nurses had advised them that we did not see the reason for yet another forty-eight hours. I had asked that they be prepared to explain to us exactly what they anticipated discovering in the next forty-eight hours about our mother's future that we didn't know now.

As we waited, we thought about how uncustomary we were: so many of us, so many of us articulate and unwilling to passively accept the controls imposed on us, so clearly educated about our mother's wishes and the institutions that were structured toward neglect of those wishes. I found myself feeling compassion for the physicians, who were equally caught in these forces, apprehensive about dealing with frightened and insistent families and threats of litigation. "We're the only country that openly calls our health care delivery system an industry," I shared with my family. "It creates a strange scenario, and motivates for profit and control rather than for compassion and care." We were living this dissonance. Human suffering turned into a power exchange among people with diverse interests. It reminded me of the workshop I was missing, the book contract I had not yet signed.

The physicians arrived. Apprehensive, they did not sit down but stood at the door. Mom's physician introduced the neurologist and shared with us that he had consented to a negotiation where forty-eight hours for both would be the first forty-eight hours. It seemed strange at best that this woman's life ending was about whether two physicians could share the same forty-eight hours. I had asked the nurses earlier where the concept of forty-eight hours came from— whether it was customary practice, or hospital policy, or an action of their ethics committee. They noted each physician had his or her own beliefs, that the hospital had no policy, and that the ethics committee was virtually powerless and dealt primarily with extra-ordinary cases, Mom not qualifying for this status.

The neurologist gave a brief report confirming that there was only minimal brain-stem activity that might sustain some vegetative function. He then said nervously, "I'm sorry I'm standing here, like I'm lording it over you." I noted, as the family spokesperson, that we had placed chairs for each of them and that we had hoped that they would sit with us and discuss the situation. He responded, "Oh, I couldn't do that—then [my mother's physician] would be lording it over me." We were stunned. It was supposed to be funny, but we could only marvel that the dominant power relationship between these colleagues could intrude into this difficult situation.

The nurse who had been our primary advocate was standing in the corner near the chairs observing us, there to give us support. She was overtly startled and shamed by the physician's comment and moved quickly to one of the chairs, saying, "Well, I'll sit down with you!" with perhaps too much intensity. None of us missed the gesture, knowing how she was trying to smooth over the insensitivity of the comments, and all of us were grateful. I then carefully explained to the physicians what Mom's wishes had been about extraordinary measures, how she had negotiated her living will with each of us, how strongly she felt about this, and how concerned we were that we honor this. I noted that all of us were in clear agreement about this. We then collectively affirmed this, hoping that the physicians would be more responsive if we removed any uncertainty they felt about this large group of humans attending to one patient. The risk of litigation seemed as powerful as Mom's wishes, indeed more powerful. They said they would take Mom off the ventilator the next morning.

We had a long night, then convened in the morning, went back in and prayed with her again, then left so that no one would have to watch the struggle between forced mechanical breathing and the effort toward independent breathing. We realized too that she might die thus, abruptly fighting to breathe, having lost the artificial support. None of us would be with her, and she would merely experience abrupt deprivation. We were all uncomfortable with this. The nurses noted that they thought she might survive for a while and that the transition off the ventilator could be traumatic, so we should wait outside. By now we trusted them explicitly, so we did as advised.

It was time to negotiate to make sure the other "doors" for Mom would be kept open, so I met with the doctor alone to ask these questions. We concluded that meeting with all of us had proven overwhelming to him. The nurse who had been so supportive in the large meeting had positioned herself with us, and I told the physician I wanted her there. I clarified each of the "doors" and made sure they were all open, made sure all comfort measures were being taken, pain control managed, and that there would be a do-not-resuscitate-or-intubate order written. He was weary of us by now, I think, and said, "There is no need to write this; I will be here and I will make sure that no one will intubate or cardiovert her."

I pointed out that he couldn't possibly be there all the time, and someone might not know the order. I asked him again to write it, and he refused a second and third time. As he walked away, the nurse put her hand on my arm and said, "You did a great job; he's not real accustomed to this situation, so you're helping him learn, too." I protested: "But I didn't get him to write the order; what if something happens and we can't stop someone from coming in and trying to cardiovert her?" She smiled warmly, "Oh, but they are written orders. I was standing here the whole time and heard the decision, and I need to record it." Gratitude swept over me, and relaxation.

Mom lived through Monday, struggling for air at first, then slowly relaxing into a gradual pattern of the respirations we all knew as the ones of a woman with asthma. She lived through Monday night, and Tuesday dawned with her status unchanged, though her respirations seemed to have slowed some. Her physician arrived that evening, acknowledging that we had tried again to reach him on Tuesday. He said nervously, "I thought she had died already." I was startled by his comment and realized that he too knew that she indeed had no chance of survival. Yet he had instituted the extraordinary measures despite her wishes. I also realized how hard it was for him to accept her death, and how painful it was for him now to realize that he had "trapped" her exactly where she said she did not want to be.

We kept vigil, reminisced, and tried to make real the changes in our lives we were collectively facing. Mom seemed more physically relaxed all day Tuesday, yet something seemed not complete, undone. We talked among ourselves. My oldest brother noted that a friend he had called asked if we had assured Mom that we would not let any-one cardiovert her again, hurt her again, keep her from leaving if she was ready to go. Tuesday night I reflected on this a long time, and by Wednesday morning I knew that we had not yet done for Mom all that we needed to do so she might have the death she wanted.

Mom was a religious woman, and I knew that she would only leave if surrounded by prayer. Mom loved music, and she would appreciate good music to leave with. But most of all, I believed that my brother's friend was right: we had not yet assured her that she would not again be cardioverted. I came to the hospital with a firm resolve, a tape recorder with tapes, and a certainty that surprised me. My two sisters and one of my brothers were there, having done the night vigil, and we slowly began to convene for another long day. I talked to my older brother about my ideas, and he selected some Psalms to read to Mom. I put Pachelbel's Canon in D on the tape player and turned it on. My brother spoke first, and then I took my turn, telling Mom that if she were ready to go and worried about them forcing her to come back, we had taken care of that. I said that no one would try to do that, that we would stop them, and that there were always several of us here, that we would not let anyone hurt her, she could go whenever she was ready and she would be permitted to go peacefully. My younger sister took her turn after me.

I had believed that these were the people she most needed to hear this message from and so had planned to simply go on reading Psalms and changing tapes as needed. Clearly, however, the messages she needed were those about the cardioversion threat. After my sister spoke to her, we could see her peacefully move, breath by breath, to more shallow respirations. I could see she was going to leave, assured of her safety. I went to get the nurse, came back in, and watched her quietly and peacefully breathe her last three breaths. I looked across the bed at my older brother and realized that he had just seen his first death. Later, he confirmed this. "It is the best you will ever see," I responded. She had died as she would have liked to die, but we had negotiated our way to that place; it had not been given to us, and we had done so at a very uneven table.

We, her children, find peace in the safe passage we sought for her. We have mourned and cried, laughed and sung fine songs as we honored the close of her life. We have remembered, and will continue to remember. I believe, reflecting back, that this passage taught me better than most life lessons why I had learned to negotiate at an even table. "You midwifed Mom to her death," my brother observed. I reflect on that often, the good fortune of that fact, and am grateful that I learned what I learned in all those visits to uneven tables.

There are many books I'd like to write. Mom's dying journey reinforced for me that this was the one to write now. I hope that what you learn as you read this book will bring some richness into your life, just as the lessons described here have brought richness into my life and the final chapter in the life of my mother, and we who shared in her journey toward death.

Part One

Creating the Context for a Dialogue

1

Initiating the Dialogue

Like inchworms measuring the marigold, we humans are slowly edging ourselves through a millennium experience. People who like to articulate their perceptions of this progression reflect individual propensities toward optimism, indifference, or despair. These combine to unveil a collective sense of the times, and the conflicts we feel about the times. The dialogue initiated in this book is embedded in these times.

Whether we are concerned about the small and large wars among nations, the destruction of the ecosystem, the decline of civility, the escalation of violence in our communities, the impact of stress in our jobs, or the struggles we each experience in our families and our intimate relationships, we all face conflict. Most of us would like to resolve our conflicts a bit more creatively. Thus, in one way or another, we turn to conflict resolution for aid, and perhaps for hope.

No human device provides all we might hope for. Each is flawed in the same way we humans are flawed, reflecting our limitations and sometimes perpetuating them. Conflict resolution is no different. It is a valuable but limited human device. The discovery of limits inevitably emerges from the lived experiences of those who test such a device. Since this book invites you to a dialogue about a specific limit of conflict resolution, it seems appropriate to first describe my vantage point as the author.

Every book approaches its topic from a given vantage point. This may be stated or unstated. I have elected to state mine, to the best of my ability, with some degree of candor. This decision comes from years of reading books written by people who do not state or acknowledge their vantage point and sometimes even try to hide it.

Unacknowledged vantage points are often a source of conflict or confusion. Frequently authors are unable to differentiate their vantage point from those of others because they genuinely believe that their vantage point is the only available or valid one. They may also be a bit anxious about their vantage point. They may feel that others may challenge or disagree with it. If they really need it to be the only valid one, this can be pretty frightening for the author.

I have a distinct advantage. I know that this is only my vantage point. I do, however, think it is a meaningful one and have learned that it can be useful to others. I think this with enough conviction that I have taken the time to write a book about it. But I do not need it to prevail. I am hoping to start a conversation, not elicit agreement or win an argument. I am certain that others will have myriad ideas that will enhance what I have to say. I think some suggestions will clarify my thinking more, and I know that this is to my advantage. If I say the things I have to say as clearly as I can from my vantage point, others might better connect with my worldview, and that will also be to my advantage. As you read further in this book, you will discover that this is just one of the advantages that emerge from learning how to constructively be at an uneven table.

On Getting Situated

A vantage point is really a metaphorical device for clarifying a position; as Einstein revealed, what I see depends on where I'm at. In this sense, my position is clarifying. It has been my experience that actually the only place I can be is where I am, and being clear about where I am enables me to better understand where other people are. But I am somewhere, and that location makes a difference.

From a vantage point, I can survey the terrain called "reality." As with any other unique human, some things will capture my attention more than others; I will elect to focus on some things more intently. I also may completely fail to focus on some realities. I further bring my personal set of characteristics to the terrain called "reality," and these serve as lenses and filters, in much the same way as one "sees" through a camera lens.

As I describe my vantage point, both the choices of focus I have made and the lenses and filters I use are important. They are so intertwined that distinguishing one from the other is a bit artificial, but I will attempt to do so here for purposes of clarity. My focus leads to a set of premises that have shaped this book; my lenses and filters are the personal characteristics that have provided tonal hues to my observations and my descriptions of what I have seen.

Sharpening the Focus: The Premises of This Book

The most compelling premise of this book is that the resolution of human conflicts is a moral enterprise that is the responsibility of every human. To not pursue the creative and constructive resolution of human conflict is to knowingly and deliberately further divisiveness and the harms such divisiveness creates. Norman Cousins, in a legacy to the culture he so valued, wrote a book shortly before he died called *The Pathology of Power* (1987), an analysis of our nuclear arsenals and their dangers. His final words in that book capture this moral imperative: "Beyond the clamor of clashing ideologies and the preening and jostling of sovereign tribes, a safer and more responsible world is waiting to be created" (p. 208).

This observation points to my second premise: we humans have conflicts over many things, and we do not always engage in conflict because of dominance power concerns. This focus is important, because it points to a systematic bias that seems to pervade analyses of conflict and conflict resolution. That bias, simply stated, is an overattention to a single concept: power as control of something or someone, as dominance, as the ascendance of one's self-will. In this book, I have called this concept dominance power.

Although the propensity for pursuing opportunities to exercise dominance power is a significant human trait, if one focuses on it to the near exclusion of all others, one does not capture other dimensions of interest and importance to persons involved in conflict. Indeed, dominance power concerns tend to focus on a somewhat less evolved and more exploitative dimension of what it means to be a human. This bias tends to distort not only the analysis of conflicts but also the assumptions about the desired outcomes of participants.

Conflict resolution as a field of endeavor, laboring under this distortion, harbors a threat to its own real promise. It runs the risk of allowing room only for conflicts that fit its bias, and dismissing those who question this bias. The implicit risk is one of vacuousness, superficiality, and stasis. This benefits no one.

A somewhat more troublesome premise that flows from this is the assertion that persons who reveal these distortions and misconceptions are often dismissed and discounted because there is a vested interest in denying these issues and in sustaining current dominant power structures and assumptions. Those who wish to bring conflicts to a sound resolution, like all humans, wish to succeed, to be proven correct, just, righteous. To be confronted by one's biases can and often does evoke mere defensiveness, feigned agreement, or withdrawal, rather than an honest appraisal of the multiple realities present in a situation.

My final premise is that an unacknowledged overemphasis on dominance power leads to the persistent creation of unacknowledged uneven tables. Dominance power by its very nature assumes that some persons will dominate others. To the degree that such relationships are socially structured and sanctioned, they will be created, recreated, and reinforced during conflict resolution negotiations. Hence, conflict resolution efforts may actually serve to exacerbate conflict, supporting socially structured and sanctioned inequities based on dominance power. I believe that revealing these distortions and misconceptions is meritorious, even if not initially welcome.

One way of revealing these is to describe how people accommodate such distortions and misconceptions in ways that are either constructive or harmful. The latter unveil the costs of ignoring the problem and demonstrate how conflict resolution efforts may actually increase conflict. The former provide some avenues of exploration that may reveal a potential path out of a potential morass. This book, which emerges from the premises I have just recorded, is an attempt to engage in a revealing dialogue of this nature.

Revisiting the Premises

In preparing the second edition of this book, I revisited and reflected upon these premises. Several years of teaching and training others have actually intensified my convictions about the premises. Indeed, it seems sometimes that they were actually understated. In a culture where "power" tends to mean "power to control others," imagining other types of power seems elusive. Understanding the concept of dominance power is easy; catching oneself perpetuating it as a behavior pattern is more difficult.

I have therefore searched for mechanisms to help people imagine other kinds of power. I have further explored and refined my own definition, describing power as "life energy" in an effort to focus on the primary meaning of power: self-agency, the capacity to act, to have an influence.

What has startled me is the degree to which many people cling to a single concept of power, the one that focuses on "control over others." What is perhaps more sobering is the frequent assumption that such dominance power is actually a type of entitlement, accompanied by intense emotion when threats to this control present themselves. The response is often attacking, full of rage, sometimes vengeful. This too has become part of my dialogue with others, and in the years since initial publication of this book I have learned that open discussion about the loss of dominance power as entitlement can evoke far more destructive emotions than I might originally have indicated.

I say this primarily in the interest of honesty. Articulating the nature of uneven tables for persons who not only are unaware of their nature, but also are interested in never facing their impact has proven instructive. I think I better understand the persistence of sustaining uneven tables, not merely as habit but also as vested interest. It is one thing to negotiate at an uneven table; it is quite another to publicly reveal its nature to persons who believe themselves entitled to maintain inequity. My experiences have thus led to the addition of some heretofore unstated premises.

Uneven tables often exist because individuals have very personal vested interests in creating and sustaining them, and attach these interests to perceptions of personal entitlement. When this is the case, unveiling deliberate inequity can evoke persistent and sometimes volatile interpersonal violence. It probably needs to be said, even though it doesn't feel like good news. Perhaps it is not only a premise, but also a caveat.

Fear of this potential interpersonal violence can motivate disadvantaged persons at the uneven table to prefer conflict avoidance, to consent to compromise and adaptation, even when it is contrary to their own best interests and the interests of others. They can also align themselves with those claiming entitlement, join forces with them in one fashion or another, and then seek to sustain the status quo. This complicates the work of persons at an uneven table who have seated themselves in the interest of creative conflict resolution. This too is both premise and caveat.

Perceived entitlement counts, especially when it is threatened.

Acknowledging the Lenses

In 1994, I noted that in addition to these premises, my vantage point as the author of this book is also shaped by who I am, by my specific traits and characteristics. Several of these are germane when one considers negotiating at uneven tables, when one acknowledges the overattention in this country to dominance power, and when one attempts to make distinctions between constructive and harmful models of conflict resolution. My vantage point is that of a person who has been on "both sides" of the imbalanced distribution of dominance power, one who has made the errors of both sides, and one who has had the opportunity to experience and value the strengths and opportunities of both sides.

I am a person with European-American, Judeo-Christian, Greco-Roman roots raised in a culture dominated by these exact perspectives and values. They are familiar to me, and I grew up assuming not only that they were the right ones, but that they were virtually the only ones, all others being distortions or errors. More specifically, my roots are German American, Roman Catholic, and Midwestern United States. Even writing this makes me feel sort of stereotypically wholesome, like homemade bread and the Fourth of July.

I am also a woman, raised in a culture dominated by values of forced gender structuring, where being a woman was largely that which was not being a man. I was taught that a man was a superior entity in what the culture valued most: agency and control. My life experiences and education have been largely dominated by masculine perspectives—which are rarely called that. I am now fifty-eight years old. During my lifetime, I have experienced cataclysmic changes about what it means to be a woman in the United States, and therefore inevitably in what it means to be a man. These changes seem to me to have been, until recently, more actively initiated by women than by men.

I am a professional academic, enjoying all the status and privileges awarded the scholar in U.S. society. I have significant opportunities to know, learn, and discover and view these as beneficial and personally enriching. I take great pleasure in both the teaching and the creating elements of academe and believe I am involved in worthwhile work.

I am a professional nurse, embracing membership in one of the most gender-structured, systematically exploited, and oppressed occupational groups in the United States. I believe nurses engage in one of the most profound services given to humans. I take enormous pride in knowing I am a member of this cadre of powerful, caring persons who truly make a difference in the quality and meaning of human existence. I also believe few occupational groups have experienced so much institutionalized and socially sanctioned injustice.

The years between the first and second editions of this book have seen cataclysmic change in health care in the United States. As I am writing, the most serious nursing shortage in my career is unfolding. Current studies demonstrate that the "downsizing" of hospitals during the 1990s has shortened patient length of stay, keeping only the very sick as patients, while concurrently introducing massive layoffs of the registered nurses who care for these very sick patients. This process, variously described as the reengineering or redesign of health care, purported to improve the health care delivery system. The resultant layoffs, a cost-saving "quick fix" often neglectful of the impact on the well-being of patients, created even more untenable working conditions for the nurses who remained. Many nurses, both those who were retained and those who were not, simply left nursing.

Recently, the impact this "reduction in force" had in terms of errors, accidents, and harm to patients has been documented. Hospitals simply have too few professional nurses, with staffing often well below safety levels. Increasingly, patients cannot be admitted to hospitals because there are no nurses to care for them. The result is poorer, less safe, and often more insensitive patient care. Fewer people wish to be nurses, looking at the career patterns that seem inevitable: "mandatory" overtime, excessive workloads, undervaluation of contribution, chronic discounting of expertise, inadequate pay for responsibilities assumed, limited job satisfiers. Nurses who were "downsized out" are certainly not interested in returning to this chaos. The table has become more uneven than it was in 1994.

I note this because it has increased my sense of urgency about what I have to say here. It is an urgency that will increasingly be experienced by every person who is hospitalized in the United States. This "update" seems noteworthy.

As my comments indicate, the conflicts in these "givens" of my life are substantial, but the conflicts themselves have taught me a great deal, often through trial and error, with more mistakes than I can at this point chronicle. I have learned to value these conflicts, however, because they have called forth in me a commitment to courage, self-honesty, and learning that I might not have acquired without the conflicts. They have sometimes fatigued me but have not permitted me to indulge in prolonged periods of sloth. They have stretched and thus enriched me—even the ones that enraged or frustrated me the most. And they have given me opportunities for personal growth and fulfillment that I might not have known had I lived a more naturally harmonious set of givens.

Thus, my vantage point in writing this book is that of a person awarded some privileges due to my membership in dominant cultures and groups, and not awarded some privileges due to my lack of membership in dominant cultures and groups. What living fifty-eight years has taught me is that both memberships have been invaluable, and both, ultimately, in many respects, are advantageous. What teaching others about this dual membership has taught me is that awareness comes slowly, often painfully, sometimes angrily. For many it has seemed like a flowering, a quantum leap of sorts, a thing of great beauty and joy. For some, it is a terror-filled discovery. For a few, it is a cause for rage.

It has become apparent to me that this dual membership has distinct advantages and makes me both intellectually and operationally bimodal, bilingual, and bifocal. Over time, I have learned that it has eventually led more often to being multimodal, multilingual, and multifocal. Once one is divested of the illusion of a belief in "the only right way," the doors open to a myriad of ways, each with some truth and some distortion, all enabling clarity. Thus, while there are substantive discomforts in dual memberships, there are also remarkable gains in terms of insight, education, opportunity, and personal growth.

Over time, this has developed in me a greater facility in seeing many sides of an issue. Indeed, eventually it has led me to be unable to do otherwise in the interest of personal integrity. It also makes it much harder for me to believe that I have the right answer, or that anyone else does. Finding meaning, discovering that which is of worth, becomes a searching process where everyone's help is welcome. Staying in dialogues becomes a priority.

This vantage point is obviously only one version of dual membership. It is, like most others, if explored creatively, useful. It can further dialogues across historically untraversed chasms between individuals and groups. Years of practical experience, both successes and failures, can refine these skills. I have thus learned not only what works but what doesn't work. This book is an attempt to share what these diverse experiences have taught me, to make them useful to others confronting the anomalous situation of being equal and unequal at the same time. It is my personal belief that this includes everyone.

Further Refining My Lenses

When I first wrote about uneven tables, I was struggling to describe experiences that were as real to me as my hands, yet often denied as real by others. I have since had hundreds of dialogues that assure me many share these experiences. This validation has been very positive for me, and I acknowledge this with gratitude.

I have also learned that my acknowledgment of the subtle impact of uneven tables on conflict resolution efforts seems congruent with some larger set of global shifts toward heightened communal consciousness, and it encourages me to have so many companions on the journey. These like-minded persons are a balm to me, as I try to live out my understanding of the challenge of intellectual integrity. I am grateful for their presence in my life.

Conversely, I am increasingly sobered by the violence, rage, and sense of impotence that seems to take possession of persons habituated to the advantages of uneven tables when that advantage diminishes. As these shifts continue, those with a deep sense of entitlement seem increasingly troubled. It warrants mentioning.

Observing persons who have a sense of entitlement has led me to explore some further dimensions of this topic that shed light on the impact on the entitled facing the loss of entitlement. These topics include the high cost of oppression for the oppressor, the depth of what I call the "victim-think" of the oppressed, the intensity of attachment to the secondary gains of conflict avoidance, and the impact of the shadow side of human personalities when that shadow is denied and projected onto others.

Perhaps for me the most interesting of these new explorations focuses on those persons at uneven tables who, to deal with their disadvantage, have embraced the values and behaviors of the advantaged in a derivative and imitative fashion. The "false entitlement" assumptions attached to such imitation of oppressors can make these persons even more violently opposed to change than the original oppressors were.

These added lenses have led me to begin to write a second book that builds on but goes beyond this one. It seemed important here to acknowledge that these additional lenses frame the pictures I now study and call my life, and the changes I have made in the second edition of this book.

2

Approaching an Uneven Table

When negotiating a conflict, on one's own behalf or that of others, a site of negotiation is created, a table. Each person brings to that table a set of personal givens, including some I've just identified in describing my vantage point. There are myriad others. In a culture where some persons are viewed as appropriate to be at a given table, others are implicitly viewed as inappropriate. The latter group often struggles over time to get to the table, to be part of the negotiation.

It is often difficult to accept the fact that getting to the table assures nothing at all. Uneven tables are a problem. It is my contention that this reality has not, however, been adequately explored. There are many potential avenues of exploration available.

I may find that I am permitted at the table, indeed, even invited to the table, but am unaware of all the implicit and explicit assumptions that guide being at the table. Everyone at the table may communicate an assumption of parity among participants, but the emotional acceptance of such parity may not be established, either consciously or unconsciously. As a young academic, I was often the only woman in committee meetings. A singularly gracious gentleman once assured me that he was really pleased to see a woman on the committee because all the other members were so ugly to look at and I provided a more "comely vision." Deliberations on health care teams where nurses are invited to participate often involve the nurse "giving input" so important decisions can be made elsewhere, by others.

I may find that I do not have the skills to be at the table, or the assumptions about these skills do not extend to me. These can include devices of language, topic, symbolic face-saving gestures, or the uses of humor. I was once involved in an initiative to bring together the efforts of two academic committees seeking common goals but locked in competing agendas. I was the only woman on either committee. The first meeting involved a luncheon where we could get to know one another better. The ritual to achieve this was an in-depth discussion of baseball, both yesterday's game and the season in general. Although I knew some things about both, every contribution I made was ignored until I quit trying. The other participants assumed that I knew nothing about baseball, and thus my comments virtually never registered with them and only created dissonance rather than enhancing communication.

I may find that I am not at the table for the same reasons that others are at the table. Nurses, who have over time grown accustomed to the fact that they continue to practice nursing for the deep personal satisfaction it gives them, often do not negotiate from a premise of trying to control others. Care of others teaches nurses that trying to control the patient is the most useless of agendas. Hence, they often find themselves negotiating on the patient's behalf and being perceived as attempting to control the patient. The fact that someone might elect to simply negotiate as an advocate for another is not recognized as a reason to be at the table.

Reasons for being at the table often differ, and often few if any persons at the table consciously know all their reasons for being there. Negotiations can unveil further motives, switching from patient welfare to face saving or defending one's decisions. These shifts can be rapid, unexpected, and disorienting. Effectiveness diminishes under such conditions.

I may discover that I really do not want to pay the price of a seat at a table, either in personal responsibility or in compromised integrity. Sometimes I may be invited to the table precisely so that I can absorb responsibilities others choose to evade. I may be invited to the table so others can attempt to coopt me and thus silence my concerns or issues. I may find myself the token woman or man, or the token representative of an occupational, ethnic, or religious group, seated largely to silence my constituencies. Later, I may find I am a handy scapegoat.

I may discover, finally, that I do not know when, how, or why to leave the table. If I have fought very hard to get to the table, my leaving has a heavy burden attached to it. If I represent others who would be unrepresented, I may fear that I have failed these others. I may not be able to ascertain why I shouldn't be at the table anymore, even though I feel I should leave. I may stay too long, harming myself and others. I may leave too early, or too late, or with a lack of clarity.

These are just a few of the ways that I can misread the table, that I can struggle to get to the table, and once there, find myself ill-equipped to negotiate. Conflict resolution is a human device. It is also a complicated process. It is as useful as the honesty and courage brought to bear in the process allow. Multiple vantage points can help enhance potential outcomes.

The insights in this book are not the only ones or the best ones. They are, however, ones that are largely missing in the existing exploration of conflict resolution. It is my hope that they will augment, enlarge, and enrich the insights already available.

A Story

Timothy was dying. His translucent skin stretched over bones that charted a tiny skeleton that made me feel like I was viewing a miniature x-ray. His tummy gaped open from surgical incisions that would not heal. Born with so many anomalies that he had no chance of survival, he was being fed through a tube directly into his stomach because he couldn't swallow. But he couldn't digest food either, and he was starving to death. Life seemed so bereft for this three-week-old mystery. Yet he had amazing sparks of normal. He had a tremendous sucking reflex and had sucked and gnawed on his tight little fists until they were raw with abrasions.

"He needs a pacifier!" The thought emerged spontaneously, clear logic from my limited wisdom as a naïve twenty-one-year-old student nurse. Timothy had been stretching my limited coping abilities, and this insight proved to be no exception. I went to the head nurse to ask for a pacifier for this small mite of humanity with so little pleasure in his short life.

She looked at me with that bland stare of a person grown too accustomed to pain, and told me that the hospital didn't stock pacifiers. So I volunteered to go buy one. She was clearly not pleased. She pointed out to me that none of the infants used pacifiers, that they were considered orthodontically and psychologically unwise. I tried to cajole. I failed.

I went to look for my instructor, knowing that she would not welcome my arrival. An hour earlier we had shared the trauma of my first injection. I had protested that I would like to start with a patient a bit less tragic. The thought of sticking a needle into Timothy was more than I could endure. She was firm and advised me I would have to get over these kinds of reactions. We selected a tiny needle normally used for a shot beneath the skin. I was so nervous I broke the glass vial that contained Timothy's medication and cut myself. It took a while to clean up the bleeding, draw up the medication, and nervously find a spot on Timothy's bottom where we could imagine a small muscle should have been developing. I had done it, but it had been an awful experience.

I had a hunch that assigning me to give my first injection to Timothy had been a punitive gesture. The instructor was not pleased with my impertinent questions, my willingness to challenge everything, my general lack of docility. She was consistently troubled by my unwillingness to learn that nurses were to be compliant and submissive. Her anger was always palpable. I dreaded facing her, but I dreaded failing to give Timothy some pleasure even more. So I found her and made my proposal. She consented, but I vaguely sensed this was going to be one more opportunity to be shown my limits.

I approached Timothy's parents, who were several years older than me, and explained to them that since their baby had such a healthy sucking response, he was injuring his fists trying to find something to suck on. This was their fourth child, and he had caught them unaware. They were accustomed to healthy babies; the truth of mortality appeared to have visited them prematurely. I never quite felt we were in touch, but then they seemed not to be in touch with anyone, even with one another. Their pain was as complex and compelling as Timothy's plight.

They consented and thanked me for trying to do something to make Timothy feel better. I was pleased with myself, feeling I had given them something concrete to focus on, something positive. They clearly liked the idea that something nice could happen to Timothy. He had sustained three unsuccessful surgeries, and they had been advised that now they would simply have to wait for him to die.

When his doctor came for rounds, I approached him to make the same request, as advised by both the head nurse and the instructor. He became agitated with me and said he could not consent to giving Timothy a pacifier. He said that if you give children pacifiers, they become dependent on them. I pointed out that Timothy had only a few days to live.

I sensed his anger and disapproval of me. I felt my anger and disapproval of him. "I have eight children. Not a one of them ever used a pacifier!" he shouted.

He refused to consent to my request. My anger intensified. I gave my short lecture on normal growth and development, sucking reflexes, and the right to modest pleasures as one dies. I told him I had the parents' consent. He was not pleased that I had approached the parents. Communications with the parents were, he believed, his domain. My job was to support his decisions, whether I liked them or not. We sparred a bit longer, and he gave in, in part, I think, because I was so tenacious. I triumphantly went out and purchased a pacifier.

Four days later, a nurse who shared my commitment to giving Timothy a pacifier called me at home. Timothy had died. In the four days between that pacifier purchase and his death, I had replaced the pacifier three times. It had been confiscated, or lost, according to the report of a night nurse who agreed with the doctor. It was a tough fight giving Timothy even a little pleasure.

That one pacifier split the unit. Some nurses supported the measure, some did not. My stubborn forcefulness had not really succeeded, or had at least only succeeded in part. My instructor was angry with me, the physician was displeased, and the nurses took various positions and acted accordingly. The family was left trying to make sense of this uproar.

Timothy was the first patient of mine to die. I mourned for days. I can never see a pacifier without thinking of him. I think not only of that small creature dwarfed by my large hands, but of the conflict this one need of his created. It has taken me years to understand that my lack of ability in negotiating this need was both a success and a failure. I did not realize that I was negotiating at an uneven table. Even had I known, I would not have known how to do it constructively.

3

The Roots of Our Distortions

The most fundamental insight, the starting point of this book, involves recognizing the imbalances we create in our perception of reality when we overemphasize dominance power. This asks a lot of you as a reader, since our social systems reinforce this overemphasis. You might best approach this dialogue by suspending judgment until you have read the last page and reflected on it all.

Before we were confronted with the threat of polio, cancer, or AIDS, we neither focused on these diseases nor worried about them. Once we recognized they existed, we were able to see new options and select new behaviors and new outcomes. This book is written as an invitation to experience the imbalance of dominance power in that spirit, with the same increases in freedom potentially emerging from the insights. I don't really want to experience any of these diseases, but denying their existence makes me more vulnerable than I would be otherwise. We cannot make choices until we understand our options.

This focus on choosing points a veiled arrow back to a prior assertion: this book assumes a moral enterprise as a dimension of human existence. It also points to the primal dilemma of a person seated at an uneven table: the need to exercise moral efficacy in an environment that may—indeed, that often will—define the situation as free of moral deliberation. If the person is viewed as lacking dominance power, the negotiation may further assume that he or she cannot function as a moral agent.

Distortions of Democracy

This dilemma is profound, albeit understandable in the context of the dominant culture in the United States. In this culture, choice has a commonly held definition based on a collective concept of personal freedom within a democracy. In the United States, the definition of democracy is rooted in Greco-Roman conceptions and assumptions.

Democracy emerged from a profound vision of the human person's potential for self-responsibility within a social system. It was, however, also conceived in distortion. The founders of democracy, both Greek and early American, crafted their vision as germane to only a select group, as a model of privileged dominance. Democracy was not only a possibility, but also a responsibility for some humans, though not all humans. Those outside the boundaries of privilege were perhaps to be cared for, protected and sheltered, but they were clearly not capable of self-responsibility. Rather, they were called on to serve those who directly enabled the democracy.

Greek culture viewed women as less than human, embraced slavery, destroyed unwanted children, and used war as a problem-solving device. These roots, both historical and mythical, are difficult to deny. Thus, democracy laid claim to a compelling vision of human potential for self-governance but denied this privilege to many. Less overtly, it denied the impact such a choice would have on both the privileged and the unprivileged. This set of propositions undergirding the democracy provided a definitional frame for those who had as well as those who had not.

Those people ineligible for citizenship were confronted by a sobering dilemma. If they agreed to the social definition, they in effect made it come true, both sustaining and perpetuating the claims of the privileged. If they disagreed with the social definition, they proved that they were defective, for they were incapable of recognizing the truth, rightness, and justice of the existing definitions of reality. Once more, they supported the claims of their "superiors" through their rebellion. This fundamental dilemma can easily be recognized by anyone seated at an uneven table.

I like to believe it is obvious, but it seems rarely so, that the roots of democracy were predicated on the assumption of "inferiors" as part of the social network.

We seem less able to confront this assumption of the presence of "inferiors" among us today. We assume someone to be governed, someone to dominate, someone over whom one would exercise power, albeit in their best interest as perceived by those in power. We want to believe we are making careful and wise choices for those incapable of self-governance. We seem least of all able and willing to honestly confront the fact that we seem to need "inferiors" in order to feel adequate, to have someone to dominate. We have also required of "inferiors" that they accept and sustain their inferiority. To do otherwise is to threaten the "democracy."

These are deep roots, both culturally and emotionally. We do not question or explore them comfortably. We will not shift them readily. Hence the illusion that we who live in democracies set only even tables, or actually seek to do so, is rarely confronted. Rather, we have created democratic structures that assume an uneven table, and perpetuate it. This is a critical insight for those seated at uneven tables. For the privileged, there is the threat of being disabused of illusions and claims to entitlement; for the unprivileged, there is the dilemma of cooptation, withdrawal, or discounted rebellions.

Hence, before even exploring this topic, it is useful to clarify for yourself your stance concerning these distortions. The clearest stance is simple: I am a moral agent. You have to assert this clarification at least to yourself, knowing that you may sometimes be the only person at the table that affirms that assertion. The consequences of this assertion are substantial. As a moral agent, I am not only able to do good, but, by claiming my own moral agency, I take responsibility for the failures of my moral agency. This asks a great deal of me, and of you. It may be why the whole topic is so unexplored. As Robert

Pirsig (1991, p. 430) frames it, "The most moral activity of all is the creating of space for life to move onward."

The other side of this assertion can be equally troublesome: everyone else at the table is a moral agent, whether they are aware of or accept this reality or not. Freedom of choice really is freedom of choice, even if it means that I choose to abuse or exploit others or choose to deny my self-responsibility. Indeed, even where others manifest severe limitations, the choosing is still intact. We can argue that we could make choices for others, but the implicit omnipotence and arrogance are readily apparent. Less apparent may be our need to view someone else as inferior to shore up a diminished sense of personal adequacy. I may choose to sustain those who I perceive as inferior in their inferiority simply to assuage my own limited sense of self-worth. We do not escape making errors in this process; we tend to exacerbate the ones we are already making.

Distortions of Privilege

When I read Eastern philosophical treatises, I intuitively realize that the culture I live in is very attracted to an illusion of "the right answer" or "the one final best true thing." This illusion is tough to sustain, of course, because it requires denial of the human condition. It also emerges from our interest in dominance power. Dominant cultures, groups, and individuals tend to need to "be right or superior" to sustain that dominance.

This cuts persons off from other vantage points. They are so busy protecting their own vantage point that they fail to openly explore those of others. This seems to me to be a tragic error in judgment, as it inevitably leads to the denial of some dimensions of our collective reality. It tends to assume that other vantage points either don't really exist or lack validity or worth. Thus, persons who hold dominant power are often distorted or limited in their thinking and judging. Perhaps more disturbing is the fact that they fight to sustain their blindness and resist the opportunity for growth and self-expansion through the discovery of the other through the eyes of the other. This diminishes everyone.

Conversely, those who do not have dominance in a culture or subculture can feel disallowed, silenced, dismissed, or ignored. If they are too persistent, outspoken, or rebellious in their refusal to accept the dominant viewpoints, the outcomes can be even more damaging to them. They may also elect to despair and withdraw, or to subvert the dominant culture in violent, manipulative, or covert ways. This too diminishes everyone.

The tendency, when reflecting on these virtual truisms, is to assume that the only persons who experience these outcomes are those who are involved in dynamics where dominance is a manifestation of power over others. Dominance can also be a manifestation of intelligence, fear, love, greed, compassion, lust, vision—any of a myriad of human traits that can become ascendant in a given conflict. Thus, while these dynamics tend to occur around issues of power, they are also the stuff of uneven tables, involving negotiations about other human dimensions, such as nurturance or critical thinking.

This "mental trap" of reducing all discourse to issues of dominance power is indeed a recurring theme in this book. It will perhaps seem tedious to you as the reader that I keep bringing this up, but it is the message in this book, and my voice seems a small one in contrast to the culture at large.

Perhaps nothing captures the troublesome nature of this imbalanced view about dominance power as well as the discovery by social scientists that oppressed groups tend to imitate the oppressor. This has at least two germane dimensions. One is imitating the oppressor in the hope that one will then gain a share in the resources of the oppressor, and therefore feel less oppressed. The other is more subtle, and leads oppressed people on a circular path where the very thing they oppose they then immediately recreate. If the central focus of a culture is dominance power, every oppressed person would reasonably seek dominance power, so they could then transact the very wrong they reject. The self-defeating nature of this for humans as individuals seems relatively self-evident.

Distortions of Disadvantage

While those who come to uneven tables privileged, or imitating those who are privileged, bring one set of distortions to a negotiation, those who come from a vantage point of perceived disadvantage bring another. They may work to get to the table, yet once there find themselves unable to function. They may lack dominant culture skills, and fail to realize they need to learn them. They may evaluate events at the table from a skewed perspective, unable to understand the assumptions of those who are there with a sense of privilege. They may know that they are at the table for different reasons than others, but fail to discover the reasons and interests of these others. The pace set by those more accustomed to the table may be too rapid or intense, hence disorienting. The disadvantaged may need to leave the table and believe they cannot or should not. They may find it embarrassing to admit to any of these additional disadvantages, once at the table.

Cooptation happens. Those disadvantaged at the table may not even realize it has happened. They may honestly think they are negotiating successfully, simply because they are at the table and engaged in the dialogue of the table. Disadvantage without clarity or competence has its own costs.

Distortions of Silence

Persons who find themselves chronically seated at uneven tables, where overt dominance power is the only or central measure of reality, may have become skilled at being at such tables. They often sustain their viability under these conditions through silence—that is, not acknowledging that they are using an alternate set of insights and skills unavailable to those denying the existence of an uneven table. This silence has a certain power. Those who feel chronically disadvantaged are reluctant to let go of this power. They also do not trust this power when it is in the hands of others attending to an overt display of dominance power.

Discussing these issues thus involves a moral risk that the information will be used manipulatively by those embracing dominance power and those who imitate them. Not discussing these issues also involves a moral risk, one of perpetuating harms through silence. This brings me full circle, to the first premise of the book: resolving conflict is a moral enterprise that is the responsibility of every human; to not pursue the creative and constructive resolution of conflict is to deliberately further divisiveness and the harms such divisiveness creates.

Distortions of Pride

It is clear to me, after fifty-eight years of living, that I have made several unwise choices, that I continue to do so, and that as long as I am human I am likely to further this track record. The measure of my character and worth is not whether I have avoided making poor choices, but how willing I have been to learn from these errors in an effort to not repeat them, and how I have elected to attend to their consequences. To sustain and defend errors because I am reluctant to correct them merely deepens my enmeshment in error. To seem to not choose is also a choice, often the poorest of the alternatives.

4

Recognizing an Uneven Table

S o, what exactly are uneven tables? How do they look, and how do you know that you're at one?

The concept itself is metaphorical. It is one of several metaphors used to describe a situation of inequality. A related one in common usage is an "uneven playing field." In each, the message is that something one hopes to find even is not. I personally like the image of the uneven playing field, but it always makes me wince. As a young girl I was forced, as were my female peers, to play half-court basketball. I was so frustrated by this that I lost my enthusiasm for the sport. Later, watching my daughters' soccer teams, in deference to boys' teams, assigned to the worst fields at the worst hours with the worst schedules and referees, I revisited my childhood frustration. I could not imagine writing a book with those images present at all times. At least there are some clear images for sitting at a table that seem to apply to all humans.

And the metaphor of the uneven table is an apt one for understanding the process of conflict resolution. The table refers to the site of a negotiation, fulfilling the dictionary definitions of "a group of people assembled at or as if at a table" and "a legislative or negotiating session." In a formal process of attempting to resolve a conflict, this table is "set" by one or more negotiators, who attempt to ensure that the table is even, so that the "table" can then meet the more concrete definition: "a piece of furniture consisting of a flat slab fixed on legs." If one of these legs is too long, too short, broken, or missing, the table tilts, perhaps even collapses, and its "tableness" becomes doubtful, as does its utility.

According to the dictionary, evenness refers to something being "balanced, in equilibrium, equal, fair." This is well captured in the colloquial term "breaking even," which refers to finishing neither as a winner nor as a loser. People who come to a negotiation seeking only to win will of course find evenness a deterrent. They have to consent to this evenness in some sense, but it could result in their merely "breaking even." It is perhaps self-evident that starting out uneven would make it unlikely for everyone to break even.

It is the task of one negotiating in a conflict to increase his or her potential for success by actively structuring for an even table. A common approach is to make certain that all parties to the conflict have a seat at the table. One of the interesting variants on this is to give historically powerless players additional seats at the table. This has the interesting effect of telling all the parties to the conflict that this party is so weak that it takes two or more of them to equal a normal person. It serves to reinforce the powerlessness.

Another approach is seating people who have historically never been there, and then expecting them to successfully negotiate on their own behalf despite the sizable gap in skills, experience, and cultural training between such new participants and those who have been there for some time. In addition, in this situation, the fact that the mores, customs, and values of the group who have been there for some time will prevail is ignored, and the new participant is expected to adapt rather than change these mores, customs, and values. Indeed, the new player is considered a "problem" if this adaptation does not occur.

A Story

I once served on a statewide committee looking at maldistribution of health care services and hoping to alter this with changes in health care professionals' educational practices. There were several Native American reservations in this state. Health care needs on these reservations were profound. Historically, these needs had been easily rendered invisible, the responsibility not of the state and its citizens, but of the National Bureau of Indian Affairs. An honest effort was made to change this pattern, to invite representatives from the tribal councils to the table. They attended the first organizational meeting.

The tribal councils, of course, had a well-developed model for deliberating on conflicts: requesting all parties to speak their mind on the issue one by one and uninterrupted, in a deliberative fashion; consulting the elders; seeking guidance from spirits that might help in the conflict; reflection. The approach to conflict offered by the statewide committee was open discussion and political posturing, a tug of war among competing agendas. The tribal representatives sat silently watching, saying nothing. Later one participant commented to me privately that the American Indians were sure not going to get their fair share if they didn't participate better. No one asked them to speak their mind during this time. They would only have had the opportunity to speak if they had chosen to participate in the competition for airtime. At the second meeting, they were absent.

The negotiator in a conflict is challenged to create a table and to ensure that it is an even one. The preliminary process is designed to increase the potential for success of the actual work of conflict resolution: negotiation. Negotiation refers to an activity that is actually only one of a range of possible responses to resolving a conflict. One may have a tug of war, take turns prevailing, destroy one's opponent; there are options.

As the dictionary puts it, parties to a conflict who seek resolution through negotiation seek "to confer with another so as to arrive at a settlement of some matter" and "to arrange for or bring about through conference, discussion and compromise . . . to bring about by mutual agreement." There is an assumption that neither party will "win" or "prevail," but that some mutual outcomes will emerge that will be satisfactory to both or all parties.

These three images—table, even, and negotiation—provide a picture of the nature of an uneven table in conflict resolution. We attempt to ensure balance and fairness in a negotiation aimed at arriving at a settlement of some matter. Unevenness at a table introduces an indicator of failure in meeting that goal. Unevenness indicates that something is "unequal, irregular, or varying in quality," to quote the dictionary again. To have started the negotiation with inequality built in is to alter the entire process that follows.

An Exercise

As I was preparing this book, I asked several people to react to a draft of my ideas. One colleague wrote back, "Is all human communication conflict resolution?" This question has been worrying me ever since. We live in a competitive, litigious society. Even telling a good story can easily result in a game of one-upmanship, where the listener responds with a story that's even better, as in "You think that's bad, listen to this!"

Briefly recall and review every conversation you have had over the last twenty-four hours. Write down a list, indicating the nature of these conversations. Now, carefully review each in detail to the best of your recall. At any moment, in any of these, did a moment of competition emerge? If so, who won? If you won, did this enhance your communication? If you lost, did this enhance your communication? Was it easier or harder to continue the conversation? What did you do about it? Can you write these answers down? If not, why not?

What do you think the answers to these questions mean in terms of conflict resolution and negotiation? Were you at an uneven table?

Judging Evenness

The assurance of evenness at a table is essentially a human judgment in the practice of conflict resolution. Solutions to overt unevenness are encouraged. There is usually an honest attempt to attend to this issue, a sincere recognition of its importance. Negotiators do not set out to negotiate at uneven tables; it isn't fun and it leads to failure.

Yet negotiators attempt to meet this goal within the limits of their own human judgment. The negotiator is thus guided by both the clarity of thinking and the sustaining of distortions or misconceptions operative at any given moment of time. These can be those the negotiator brings to the task, those common in a culture, or those uniquely presented by a given conflict. As humans, we tend to succeed and survive precisely because we can accept and integrate the distortions of our given culture. It often simply does not occur to us to question them.

But the history of the species also demonstrates that there is significant variance in the acceptable distortions of various cultures, both among the members of the culture and over time. We indeed do change, though we may resist the change. Our history is in part a record of the changes and the resistances, which is how Galileo got to be famous, using a particularly dangerous approach to becoming famous.

History also shows us that the measures of equality change over time and vary by culture. Any number of measures are feasible, depending on the focus of the measuring process: age, ethnicity, wisdom, height, cunning. We can actually imagine quite a few of these measures without a struggle. Indeed, George Herbert Mead (1984), a social psychologist who talks about the power of such measuring, shows how we change our behaviors to meet the demand of measuring up.

What becomes apparent is that the judgment of evenness occurs in the mind of a negotiator in some evolutionary moment and culture along some dimension of measurement. History informs. We once negotiated in this country to improve housing for slaves. Many people didn't question slavery but wanted the living conditions of slaves bettered. We once negotiated in this country to permit women to run for political office. Before that, it just hadn't occurred to many people that women might want to, and when permitted to, many women didn't choose to do so. These issues seem anachronistic today but did not seem so in their time. These examples are useful. In each case, dominance power is assumed and operative. In neither case was the party that was the focus of the negotiation in a position to autonomously determine the outcome of the negotiation. Culture counts.

Judgments of evenness made by a negotiator also assume that the parties to the conflict—the players at the table—agree with the judgments, or, if not, view it as within their purview or ability to question this judgment. This simply isn't true much of the time. Negotiators are not omniscient and simply can't always ensure evenness. Announcing that a table is even doesn't make it so. A response that questions that assumption can often be viewed as one more ploy to keep a conflict going, or obstructionism on the part of the questioner. It can lose you your seat at the table in the future.

A Story

I once served on a committee attempting to craft a plan of action for improving access to health care for ethnic minorities. There were no minorities on the committee. This disturbed me at such a fundamental level that I kept pointing to it as a central issue. Finally, one of the group leaders turned to me and said, "You know, you're bright and articulate, but if you keep bringing that up we're never going to get this task done. I'm getting tired of hearing about that issue." The group leader was purportedly negotiating a new model of delivery designed to address long-standing inequities.

As the only nurse at the table, and invited there despite the fact that historically nurses have been systematically excluded from such deliberations, I was ill-equipped to change the process. I pointed out that I knew this fact, that indeed I was at a table from which I had historically been excluded and thus understood such exclusion. While these things were acknowledged as true, no change in group composition was pursued. When I suggested the names of possible participants, it was noted that they would confound the process. It was indicated to me that I was enough of a problem, without adding to it.

The fact is, for evenness to be assured, all parties at the table have to concur on this evenness. Much of the time this assurance is untenable. We set our tables, though, and we often don't want our decision processes questioned or modified. The conflict is troublesome enough; we hardly need opportunities to make our challenge greater than it already is. It becomes easy, even comforting, to convince ourselves that the table is even, or even enough for now.

As can readily be seen, unevenness can be further exacerbated when some people at the table agree with the negotiator's assurance of evenness, and some do not. The negotiation is contaminated before it begins. Most negotiators try to avoid this outcome and seek assurances that the table is even. This assumes that everyone who senses an unevenness is willing or able to articulate it and will be heard. Neither assumption is sound, especially as this pertains to persons historically excluded from negotiations.

Under these conditions of contamination, a strange process emerges. Some people at the table know that the negotiator and some other people in the negotiation have already reached an agreement on some judgments that either distort, ignore, discount, or deny the others' perceptions. I, for instance, find it very easy to ignore and discount persons at a table who are resisting changes I think are good and just. It is always a temptation for me to exclude them from participation or silence them when they show up. In doing so, I publicly acknowledge that I want to set an uneven table. Having done so, I contaminate the entire effort.

Sustaining Dominant Worldviews

Every culture is a network of dominant worldviews or paradigms. These guide our social living, and indeed make it possible. We all agree to stop at the red light, and fewer people get killed at intersections. We don't function well as a society without such worldviews. So we become habituated to them. They comfort us, give us predictability, tell us how to keep our life flowing along smoothly.

We can easily begin to think of such worldviews as the truth rather than as relative models. They may work nicely for us, but that does not make them a component of ultimate truth and reality. We may even become dependent on them. Driving in a country without red lights taught me that almost immediately. I had no way to find the assurance of safety.

If a negotiator begins to think of some dominant paradigms as "truth," deviants from these truths will quickly find themselves at an uneven table. Such worldviews abound: we treat everyone the same; we all agree on when to start the meeting; we are all organized; we all want coffee. Clearly, we don't treat everyone the same. If our CEO comes to the table, we act differently toward him than we would act toward the telephone repairperson. When we actually start varies with what we call starting. Socializing for ten minutes of getting comfortable with one another is "starting" for one group, and delaying the meeting for ten minutes for another. One person's organization is another's suffocation in structure and rules. Some people never drink coffee.

An Exercise

Identify a conflict that you are currently engaged in with someone, a friend, coworker, employer, partner, acquaintance. Imagine that the two of you decide to meet at a local diner to discuss the difference. Now prepare for the meeting.

First, write down exactly what you think the conflict is in your own terms. Now, write down all the issues you think need to be discussed so that you will feel like the conflict has actually been adequately explored. Now, write down the outcome you want.

Now, become the other party. Write the same three things for that person: the conflict, the issues, the preferred outcome. Compare these two lists for a while. Study them.

Now write down the real difference between you and the other person. Is it the issue you named? Does one of you come to this discussion with an "advantage"? Do both of you? What are they? Will these advantages make a difference in the outcome? Why? Do these advantages have anything to do with the original issue?

So, what are you going to do about all these new insights into this conflict?

––––––––––––

Uneven tables are more common than we like to think! I know, for instance, that I am more verbal and articulate than many people are. I know that this is an advantage. If "prevailing" is my goal, I can use this unevenness to my advantage. I can verbally outlast all sorts of folks. This points to another characteristic of an uneven table: it perpetuates dominant paradigms by discounting the deviant. Silent people are deviants in negotiation in our culture. We have accepted the worldview that says that negotiation requires forceful verbalization. Thus, my verbal behavior is not only advantageous to me, it also preserves the dominant worldview and denies the worldview that says reflection is more critical to negotiation than articulateness. Interestingly, this situation has also made me less reflective than I might have been, and therefore less effective.

Dominant Power as a Source of Unevenness

Unevenness can be further exacerbated by the assumption in our culture that dominant power is the only germane negotiable type of power. There are actually a variety of powers. French and Raven (1963) created a taxonomy of power, focusing on the nature of the influence one could have on others. One can be coercive, but can also use rewards. One can have power because of a liaison or association with a second powerful person, a particularly troublesome type of power at uneven tables. Some people have influence because others view them as the legitimate purveyors of power, or believe that they have unique expertise or positions of authority. As is evident, one may also lack influence due to the absence of acknowledged legitimacy or expertise. Such "powerlessness" is less overt and may be readily overlooked.

More recently, James Hillman provided an even more expansive look at this issue in his book, aptly titled *Kinds of Power* (1995). He identifies and explores twenty kinds of power, and thus provides a useful tool for reframing power, assisting the reader in moving away from a single definition. While he does include "control" in his list of twenty, it is perhaps worth listing the other nineteen to demonstrate the robustness of his list. They include office, prestige, exhibitionism, ambition, reputation, influence, resistance, leadership, concentration, authority, persuasion, charisma, rising, decision, fearsomeness, tyranny, veto, purism, and subtlety.

In teaching various groups about the culture's fixation on only one of these kinds of power, control, I have used Hillman's expanded taxonomy to encourage others to reframe power. In retrospect, I have repeatedly been startled at how difficult it is for others to even imagine these phenomena as expressions of power. Among our culture's fixed views, power as control has enormous tenacity. Yet, there really are multiple meanings of the word power. Even a simple dictionary definition honors the variance implicit in this term. "Possession of control, authority, or influence over others" aptly captures the concept of dominant power discussed in this book. But there are other noteworthy definitions: "ability to act or produce an effect; physical might; mental or moral efficacy; political control or influence; a source or means of supplying energy, as in motive power; and scope, comprehensiveness." Even if one were to restrict the measure of evenness to power, the options are extensive.

Assumptions about dominance power, about winning and losing on these terms, as the central aim of all parties to a conflict thus introduces substantial distortion. If evenness is assessed using this measure, everyone at the table who lacks interest in dominance power is at an uneven table. In our culture, women have been rewarded primarily for not seeking responsibility and agency. We operationalize this view by describing women as needing protection. Warren Farrell has done a superb job of explicating this assumption in his book, *The Myth of Male Power* (1993). Hence, some women may be at the table seeking protection, not exercising dominant power, or may be seeking persons with dominant power at the table to serve as protectors, seeking to exercise referent power. This confounds the process substantially.

What becomes increasingly apparent is the fact that unevenness is a complex phenomenon with substantial impact. To neglect this complexity, or attend to it superficially, is to ignore the effect it can, will, and does have on the resolving of conflicts.

The Unexamined Uneven Table

Perhaps because the skills implicit in negotiating effectively are difficult and challenging, the complexity of creating an even table and the threat of sitting at an uneven one are rarely explored in depth. As a result, the unique dilemmas sitting at such a table creates are relatively unexplored. This has several deleterious effects.

Most obviously, it keeps persons who are invited to uneven tables from accessing the opportunities presented by the offer. It inevitably limits the potential of the negotiator to succeed. It limits those seated at an uneven table from experiencing the positive potentials of conflict resolution. The eventual outcome is damaging. People begin to see conflict resolution as just one more way of sustaining existing power structures.

As a result, conflict resolution cannot present itself as a viable or trustworthy alternative to sustaining adversarialness. Perhaps more disturbing, those most committed to conflict resolution become purveyors of what they have offered to confront and solve. Persons who have had many experiences at uneven tables become skilled in recognizing them. (Some of them even write books about it.) Thus, when such persons are invited to uneven tables and are assured by a negotiator that the table is even, credibility begins to suffer. I have started this dialogue in the hope that this troublesome fact will start to be more systematically and honestly addressed and explored.

5

The Persistent Fixation on Dominance Power

Reflecting on the meaning of the use of the atomic bomb in World War II, Arthur Koestler (1978) posited that we might wish to begin renumbering our calendars, using the events of Hiroshima and Nagasaki as year one. He believed these events gave us access to a whole new insight into war and discord: we had developed the resources to annihilate the planet. He made his observation in the hope that others might join him in struggling toward more effective tools for resolving our differences.

Koestler is only one of many who have attempted to draw our attention to the need to discover new approaches to resolving conflict. Embedded in his observation and that of many others is the implicit message that to dominate without restraint is to risk damage that exceeds the threats we intended to address. To have subdued nature may mean we have merely destroyed it. Clearly, our evolutionary moment is one involved in a reappraisal of the uses of dominance power. And we are discovering that it might be in our best interest to try to solve our conflicts in some manner other than an adversarial one.

It is understandable that those who have explored the world of conflict resolution have given centrality to dominance power. To have failed to do so would have seemed unwise, since the culture itself embraces this bias. Conversely, however, an overattention to dominance power fails to capture the content or nature of many human conflicts. It serves a narrow band of human conflict; perhaps more poignantly, it helps perpetuate the underlying assumptions that create many conflicts. It reinforces the bias.

An Exercise

You are a thirty-seven-year-old Caucasian male corporate executive with a six-figure salary. You have invested wisely and are essentially independently wealthy. You and your wife are in the process of litigious divorce proceedings. You wish to quit your current job, take a more modest middle-management position with a lower salary, and put your life into raising your three children, ages seven, ten, and twelve. Your wife, who acknowledges that she finds being a parent tedious and boring, is an equally successful executive in her own small business, which you initially helped her finance.

Neither of you is involved in another intimate relationship, neither of you wishes to stay in the marriage, and both of you are angry at one another for the harms in the marriage over the years.

She sues for custody of the children and is awarded custody because she is the mother. The judge explains to you and your lawyer that women are simply better at these things and that children need their mother more than their father. He also notes that you will be taking a less prestigious position, which will be less beneficial to the children. He tells you he is a bit concerned about your stability, given your current lack of ambition and drive.

What would you say to the judge to encourage him to reconsider your request for joint custody? Is this conflict about dominant power or not? Write down your answers. If you were the judge, would you be influenced by this request for reconsideration? Why? Write down your answers.

Many of the early proponents of conflict resolution saw it as a tool of social justice, but a social justice conceived and described within the boundaries, assumptions, imperatives, and biases of their culture. The emphasis was often placed on competing parties, both or all of whom were functioning in structures controlled and maintained by persons with disproportionate dominance power and the desire to retain it. The systematic bias that emerged was one virtually fixated on dominant persons in dominant groups negotiating about dominant power. The continued sustaining of existing power structures and inequities was implicitly assumed; the goal was resolving the conflict at hand, not dramatically reconstructing social systems. Dominance power was accepted as the central premise; negotiations concluded with that premise intact.

The Durability of Dominance Power Fixations

The self-perpetuation of dominance power as a measure of worth and value is not an accident. Many who most ardently want to resolve conflicts are deeply invested in sustaining dominance power; that is why they attend to it so well. It is an important currency in many cultures and is a central one in the United States. We like being a "superpower." Presidents who start "little wars" see their approval ratings go up, and candidates who weep are dismissed as wimps.

We have contests to determine who is best at just about everything and spend disproportionate amounts of our time, energy, and national resources on contests called sports. We keep our organizational charts neat and clean so everyone knows who is in charge of everyone else.

Many people do acknowledge the maldistribution of dominance power in the United States and call it a serious problem. Most, however, do not search the arenas where they can freely give up some of their own dominance power once it is attained. Indeed, to do so is considered quite absurd by many people. One must demonstrate secondary gains through some alternative dominance power to explain such a choice; otherwise one is viewed as eccentric or perhaps disturbed. One can quit being a senator to spend time with the family, or quit being a CEO to go live by the sea, but one is asked to explain these choices. They are not inherently logical to the culture.

A Parable

Once upon a time, in a strange and foreign land, women wanted their husbands to help more with the kids. They began a major campaign. They said men should do this because it was their responsibility, too. They said it would make men better humans. They said it would be good for the kids. They said it showed justice, fairness, and general goodness of heart. Men tried changing the baby's diapers. Women said, "Hey, stand back there a minute, you're not doing that right. Let me show you how to do that. Don't you know how to do anything? That will never stay on; it will leak. I'll just do it myself!"

It really doesn't matter where and how you get your dominance power; it seems pretty hard to give it away. Dominance power appeals to our need to feel adequate, in control, worth something somewhere. It can even make us feel kind of omnipotent and invulnerable. This is all an illusion, but we tend to sustain lots of illusions, for good or ill. We may complain about the responsibilities, but we like the "right" of superiority, whatever form it takes.

Because dominance power has such a disproportionate impact on us, permeating our culture like polluted air and sentimental love songs, there are few observable alternatives that capture our attention and imagination in its stead. In the absence of alternatives, we become habituated to what we already know, have, understand.

This societal reinforcement is considerable, but the self-perpetuating energy of dominance power as a measure of value is not merely societal, cultural, economic, or political. It is deeply personal. The central currency of a society becomes a deeply embedded psychological construct. We structure our lives on its terms. We don't welcome changes in the currency distribution. They are experienced as personally disruptive.

An Exercise

You are driving in the parking lot of a large shopping mall, looking for a parking place. The store you need to get to is going to close in fifteen minutes, and the item you want to purchase is important to you. The sale ends today. You drive around in a state of growing frustration. The only open parking places you can find are ten unused handicapped spaces. You are not handicapped. If you leave the parking lot for a space further away, you won't get to the store in time. No one seems to be about to release their space. You drive by the ten empty spaces twice. Time is running out. What do you do?

Write it down. How do you feel about this? (Come on now, tell the truth. . . .) Write it down. What is the solution to this dilemma that you want to teach the next generation? Write it down. What do you think the next generation will say when you try to tell them this? Write it down.

Now, ask yourself why you didn't want to write any of this down. If you still haven't written any of it down, ask yourself if you ever will write it down. Now explain your reasoning to yourself. Now see if you've convinced yourself. How are your illusions doing today?

To acknowledge and accommodate shifts in dominance power in my culture is to experience a threat, personal and immediate, to my world, to my known predictables. I have adapted to the currency, and it gives me security to know these rules of the game. To change the distribution societally is to change the distribution of power that shapes my daily life with a partner, with children, parents, siblings. It can change how I relate to my coworkers and neighbors, my friends and social acquaintances. We count on dominance power distribution for our stability.

Fixation as Dysfunction

Despite its durability, this fixation on dominance power is dysfunctional. Using it as the standard for assessing evenness is still more troublesome. I have never negotiated at a table I believed to be even, whether as a party involved in a conflict or as a negotiator attempting to resolve one. I know that evenness is in the eye of the beholder. Eventually, unevenness rears its ugly head, in one fashion or another. We are a pretty uneven species when we accept all the ways we can "compare" ourselves to one another.

As a woman and a nurse, I know of many inequities I want addressed, but I also want a just outcome, not an increase in my dominance power. I am weary of the assumption that I am an inferior person who can be counted on to behave like a victim, but I am equally weary of the assumption that I want to victimize others in a spirit of vengeance. I am impatient with the punitive behaviors directed at supposed inferiors who do not meet the expectations of either accepting their victimhood or joining in a destructive retaliation. It is easy for me personally to document the dysfunctional nature of a fixation on dominance power.

A Story

As a dean of a nursing school, I once attempted to negotiate a collaborative educational project with a medical school administrator. My medical colleague was concerned about sustaining the current power relationship between nursing and medicine. I was interested in changing the education of the next generation of health care professionals. It was clear to me that patients were being put at risk because of the dominance power conflicts between medicine and nursing. It seemed to me that we faced a moral imperative to learn a collaborative model. Where medicine exercised excessive control or dominance and nursing failed or was prohibited from exercising professional autonomy, patient care suffered. Wherever collaborative practice prevailed, patient care was enhanced. It was not just a proposition; emerging studies supported this insight.

We met to discuss this issue. My colleague's primary agenda was to assure me that the current power relationship must be sustained, no matter how much I differed with it. The power relationship in itself was of little interest to me. I could already see that medicine's hegemony in health care was deteriorating.

My interest was in improving patient care by teaching our students to work together effectively and intelligently. No matter how many ways I stated this goal, he kept reinterpreting it as my desire to give nursing power and status. I noted that collaboration assumes colleagueship and parity. That was not the issue. The issue was patient care.

This exchange, which lasted two hours, was a series of repetitions. We were speaking two different languages. My colleague could simply not imagine a negotiation where dominance power was not the focus. In turn, my ability to convince him otherwise was limited by my definition of collaboration.

When we confront the dark underbelly of human justice concerns, of substantive moral discourse, we find that in the fabric of society many are systematically denied access to tables set for negotiations. Such persons have rarely, if ever, experienced the exercise of dominance power; they do not conceptualize it in the way that those habituated to it do, as a central dynamic. They understand it not as one who regularly exercises it but as one on whom it has regularly been exercised. The difference is substantial. If someone who has for some time assured you that you're an inferior in some dimension suddenly claims you're an equal, you don't get up the next morning and "feel" equal. You also do not become skilled at explaining your experiences to those accustomed to dominating you.

For those habituated to dominance power, it is often difficult to realize that others may have shifted their focus to alternative power models, such as personal integrity, covert manipulation, spiritual wholeness, or dependency. Such persons may also have so exaggerated the possibilities inherent in dominance power that they distort its capacity to achieve desired ends. They may not want dominance power because they do not want the responsibility and risk that accrue to those who legitimately exercise it. They may have found valuable secondary gains in not having dominance power and want to retain these advantages. Finally, they may simply find dominance power a good deal less compelling than do those who focus on it intensively.

This doesn't exhaust the list of potential dissonances resulting from a fixation on dominance power, but it begins to unveil the impact these dissonances can have. Most increase conflict over time. As an implicit bias, it requires all parties to a conflict to negotiate around a single measure of "desired parity," which is assumed to be dominance power, and further perpetuates the distortion. Where there is a blindness to such distortion, the table is by definition uneven. After struggling to get to the table, one is reluctant to then announce, "Oh, by the way, this table is amazingly uneven; are you aware of that?" It can be said, but it may not cheer anyone up much.

A Story

In my tenth year as a nurse educator, I worked in a large state psychiatric hospital housing about half of a Midwestern state's indigent mentally ill citizens, who were then required, by state law, to receive "food, clothing, and shelter when such was available." The state was of little help in furthering the hopes and dreams of quality care that I held for these patients, and it was a challenge to teach future nurses how to be creative and maximize resources for optimal gains.

I had students assigned to two different floors, each headed by the same chief psychiatrist. He determined where each new patient would be assigned on admission. He also determined staffing patterns. The fourth floor had twice as many nurses, several therapists, and several programs of care; the third floor had virtually no treatment program. Since he was rarely present on either unit, I requested a meeting with him to discuss this issue.

I presented my case matter-of-factly and pointed out that in my day-to-day dealings with the patients I saw many on each floor who could profit from treatment; I was disturbed by the maldistribution of resources. He stared at me for a brief period and then asked, "How long have you been in this business?" I gave a brief report of my work history, and was then dismissed.

I have since learned to name the look he had on his face, having seen it so many times over the years: the "you-are-introducing-issues-I-do-not-choose-to-consider-as-part-of-my-decision-making-database" look. Some conflicts are merely the result of the denial of dimensions of reality that are unattractive or troublesome to confront. Some are dismissed by merely dismissing the messenger. As a nurse, I was dismissable.

Beyond the Fixation

A directory of human conflict would describe myriad conflicts resulting from the long-term maldistribution of dominant power and an acceptance of that maldistribution. Some are even experienced as "getting even" conflicts, such as those emerging from legislation that favors a historically disadvantaged group in terms of dominant power by creating unjust disadvantages for those who have historically had dominant power. Many of these solutions assume that the resolution of the historical fixation on dominance power is to redistribute dominance power and stay fixated on it in the process. This subtle continuation of the fixation ensures further conflict.

To craft a vision for a global future that seems worth leaving as a legacy to our children and our children's children, it seems to me we need to find a way to honor values and goals that exist outside the narrow boundaries of the distribution of dominance power and that in some cases transcend those boundaries. One of the unacknowledged effects of long-term social injustice is the discovery, by those subjected to this injustice, that some things are more compelling than dominance power. In addition, some persons who have historically exercised dominance power have discovered its limits and are interested in other human agendas, but are deterred by outmoded fixations.

We may not need to feed the illusion of an even table. We may not even find this a laudable goal, since embracing illusions can be a good deal more damaging than many an uneven table. We may find it is in our self-interest to simply find constructive ways to be at an uneven table.

stroll among the shadows

on first walking texas'
east gulf coast, i found
the beach peppered with
half-moon blue balloons,
marooned men-of-war:
inflated and dead.

it took me eight years
to understand
the metaphor.

—pbk

6

Imagining Alternatives

As a youngster I was advised that if I found a prevailing norm troublesome, it was my job to find a credible alternative. This was a useful lesson. Since I clearly find our culture's fixation on dominance power troublesome, I have spent some time searching for alternative assumptions about what is of worth and value. I am recording these here since they demonstrate the possibility of discovering antidotes to our fixation on dominance power, and since they are the context within which I respond to uneven tables.

I think conflict is a dimension of the human condition, one of the givens we find waiting for us when we arrive on the planet. We also find a myriad of emotional responses to this conflict. Thus, when we try to resolve our conflicts, we often find ourselves so enmeshed in the emotions of the conflict that imagining new ways of approaching it seems like a luxury. It is not an optimal time for stretching our imaginations. Prior reflection may thus be helpful.

Accepting Mystery

When we do stretch our imaginations, we find that our minds take in that which we have not yet experienced. This transition is at first a confrontation with mystery. Mystery fascinates us. Part of what we like about mysteries is following them along and finally seeing them "solved," testing our own cleverness against the challenge. We like mysteries, but only if we can hope to solve them. Lurking mysteries without solutions remind us of our limits and can thus irritate or intimidate us. At some level, we would secretly like to have all the answers.

One of the most predictable things about books is that most authors write like they have solved a mystery, no matter what the topic. Authors feel safer writing in this manner, and it reassures readers. We cheer on the author, grateful that someone has put that nagging question to rest.

Unfortunately, I'm not able to do this with this book—or with just about anything else. Every good answer today has lurking in it the next good question. I believe that's how knowledge "is." I think that good tough questions get us closer to understanding than dogma or "right" answers. Hence, this book lacks "the-one-best-way" formulas, but it does try to honestly raise important questions and honor mysteries when they show up. Mysteries are a doorway to the profound, and lift me well beyond the simplistic repetitiousness of sparring for dominance power.

The closer I get to important truths, the more I feel paradox lurking, and it keeps me reluctant to promise more than I can deliver. Books as recipes scare me. So I am saying, "Here are some ideas to play with; see how they work for you; let me know." Accepting mystery can be an asset in creating dialogues. It also frees us to continue to learn and grow without feeding the illusion that we can know everything or the compulsion to appear as if we do.

Creating Metaphors

Cognitive scientists, over the last few decades, have revealed that we can better understand human behavior and learning by better understanding the function of metaphors. When we are trying to tell someone about an experience we've had that they've never had, we use metaphors as a bridge, as in "well, it's sort of like sliding down a razor blade naked in subzero weather." Nice metaphor. Right off, I know I'm not going to want to try this experience. The metaphor is the link between the unknown and the known.

Hence, metaphors are useful. They give us access to new things. But the new things have their own power to disrupt our lives. Sometimes the metaphor is useful, helping us to test out a new idea under somewhat safe circumstances. "Try this, it tastes just like cherry candy"—the most popular lie that parents in the United States tell toddlers taking their first liquid penicillin. This is how we try to slide in new information with metaphors.

As we soon discover, however, the new information can rise up like a tornado and cause all manner of mischief. It may not fit where I have put it, or it may not even want to be seen in the company of the other facets of my world. It may want a new place, its own place, or it may want to change everything else in the system. It can become a quite frustrating and unwelcome guest. So the metaphor is useful but can become risky on occasion.

Sometimes we tell it to settle down and quit being such a bother. Other times we try to cut a deal with it, and talk it into being the idea we had wanted it to be. Sometimes we put it in exile. Sometimes none of this works, and we must simply overhaul the system because it is unwilling to respond to even our most gracious and sincere efforts at taming.

This explains both the attraction and the danger of a metaphor when we use it to learn. It unveils the deep dangers embedded in poetry. It could let things in we never meant to let in; once there, it can create havoc. Plato knew this.

The Dream

Roofless towers of despair,
silos forged of supple stones;
I hover high, I float, I agonize.
In each, one man writhes muted solitude:
waves of shafts to infinite horizons,
in gentling winds, in invitationals.

"Fly Like an Eagle!"
I shout to deaf contortionists.

—pbk

As you may now see, the metaphor has enormous power. The metaphor can say more than the "facts." I can say I went to a family reunion or I can say I spent eight hours sorting through the human networks of my autobiography. The message of the metaphor carries more impact, says more, does more. Lakoff and Johnson wrote a book called *Metaphors We Live By* (1980), which does a wonderful job of discussing all of this at the practical human level. Among other things, they explore a key metaphor in our culture: war. In fact, I believe, with them, that it is our central metaphor.

War, of course, encompasses more than frank battle with instruments of destruction. It includes conflict, argument, contest, the clear designation of winners and losers. It is, in Carse's (1986) description of games, a "finite game." There are rules, time limits, and the victors and vanquished; when it is done, it is done.

The centrality of this metaphor in our culture is not difficult to document. When I discovered that health care advertising was identifying its "target" audience, I knew we had hit a new level of confusion. We also "conquer" disease and "attack" pathogens. We "destroy" cancerous cells using "weapons" against tumors. In a recent advertisement the American Pharmaceutical Association declared: "Cancer: It's a War. That's why we are developing 352 new weapons." We lament that AIDS is a loss of the body's "defenses" against "invading" organisms. Medicine is war.

So are advertising, business, sports, news, science, politics, economics . . . this list can go on and on. We have even mounted "wars" against poverty, drugs, violence, and AIDS. I have spent about twenty years now observing this metaphor, trying to develop a sensitivity toward it and trying to find alternate metaphors that both communicate and provide a different frame for reality. Every day I find I still use the war metaphor somewhere; every day I find myself stumbling about in the darkness failing to generate the new and useful metaphors. Even the common practice of reviewing the phases of a negotiation or mediation in conflict resolution training is described as a "debriefing," a concept whose definition is "to question or interrogate to obtain intelligence information gathered, especially on a military mission."

Further exemplars may be useful. Here are some key words and phrases that help give a sense of how we, culturally, use war as a metaphor: defend, attack, protect, strategize, outflank, line of resistance, retreat, reconnoiter, defeat, surrender, give in, fight back, conquer, vanquish, target, weapon, arsenal, win, fail, promote, prevail, humiliate, vindicate, disarm, imprison, hit the ground running, orders, shooting, fired, fired on, casualties, assault, bludgeon, squabble, mission, guard, dispute, strong arm . . . this list, too, is not exhaustive. One can replicate it by locating it where I did, in a single edition of a local newspaper. Articles included ones on the assault of a severe storm, conflicts among various organized religions, shooting a new video, and the casualties in a domestic environment.

If war is not the predominant metaphor, it is assuredly a central one. And it supports a habit of mind and heart that assumes conflict, competition, and adversarialness. It frames how we view much of life. And that, of course, has an impact. Certainly, if this is the primary metaphor used to clarify the nature of a conflict, one might understand this. If it is less consciously the primary metaphor used to resolve conflict, it is less helpful. In essence, the metaphor is sustained and strengthened because no alternate metaphor is provided to enable conflicting parties to envision a new reality.

The metaphor of war is used to explain most conflicts and their resolution. This too is not difficult to document. War and adversarialness are implicitly assumed to be the "given" of the species. The war described is usually discord based on power experienced as dominance. The solutions sustain this primary metaphor and usually only peripherally acknowledge alternate models of conflict or its resolution. In my experience, many people struggle when they try to sensitize themselves to this troublesome insight. Nonetheless, it is clear that power can also be exercised as moral agency, that some conflicts involve a struggle for self-reliance, and that human love is a powerful alternative model for conflict resolution that is rarely acknowledged.

Examining Myths

Joseph Campbell, perhaps inadvertently, has turned us all into amateur mythologists of a sort, either through personal study of his works or the effort to deal with those who have. The men's movements have evolved largely from an initial focus on mythopoetic dimensions of what it means to be a man. The women's movements reflect this same interest in the mythopoetic. Jungian psychology is grounded in such myths, and the meeting between Eastern and Western philosophies is largely a mythic conversation. Something important is emerging from these discussions about myths. They apparently have meaning for us.

Evolutionary developments like this are always a bit unsettling. One can never quite squeeze them into the right place, since they have no place. They come largely to unsettle us, to disrupt our lives and demand of us some new growth. They are rarely totally welcome. When I was a child, a myth was something used to show me the unreal, to explain to me the virtues of rationality and materialism. Much of our current meandering in the mythic seems to represent a return to our roots. We are also discovering replications or re-expressions of our myths in our history and in our daily lives.

The heightening of consciousness about myth seems often to be a function of an overall heightening of consciousness in general as an evolutionary task of the times. Imagining alternatives to various wars is one such task. We have for decades conducted a war on nature; now we advise people to be good to their mother, the earth. Imagining alternatives to armed conflict is an analogous task, and the images here may or may not prove mythic in nature. Disarmament is not the creation of peace. Often conflict resolution sustains the traditional myth of war, even as it attempts to address the limits of such myths.

I think it is important for us to begin comprehending and respecting the impact of our mythic roots. This process helps us understand the metaphors we live by; it helps us understand our own propensities and tendencies much better. There are many dimensions to this comprehension and respect. My list is not exhaustive, but bears scrutiny: religious, cultural, societal, ethnic, national, familial, and personal. All, of course, occur in a historical context. All frame our beliefs, thoughts, feelings, emotions, hopes, and dreams. They also feed and sustain these expressions of ourselves, and they are the content and the context of our daily lives. They are the templates for how we create and sustain our realities.

Some people want to create new myths. I like this idea, but I always have a lurking sense that the tougher task is confronting the ones that hold us in thrall at this time. These we live out unconsciously, sustaining and maintaining them. If we engaged in an honest scrutiny of these myths, we might begin to ask useful questions about them. We might even take responsibility for the inevitable consequences of the choices we have made. We might then imagine new choices, and find and create the myths that enable us to sustain the consequences of these new choices.

Many of the proponents of conflict resolution simply ignore the impact of the dominant myths in our culture. Yet effective resolution of conflict implicitly assumes one is willing to live with the negotiated agreement. If the agreement is contrary to some central myth in my life, I may give the veneer of concurrence to demonstrate that I am a good person, or to avoid censure, but I will not really have dealt with the conflict. I will merely have veiled it, or walled it off only to have it emerge later with some new ugly face. Suppression is not resolution. Myths revisit us, whether we invite them or not.

This country has some powerful myths. Exemplars here may be useful, though they merely skim the surface of this deep and mysterious pool. We have Greco-Roman myths in our government systems that say that equality is important, that the city-state has authority, and that slaves and women are important resources for ensuring certain outcomes (though they are not citizens). We have Judeo-Christian myths that say we are the promised people, that there is only one transcendent being favoring some people over others, that the transcendent being is a man, that this being has rules, and that he loves us by punishing us severely if we do wrong. Emerging from these myths, we have colonial myths that say it is good to claim land for yourself, that those there before you must be subdued or destroyed, taught your myths, and cared for like children. We have myths that say this is good for all aliens—that is, slaves and women, those not citizens of the state, those not like "us." We have familial myths that say a traditional American family has a certain structure, function, role, and ethic. We have personal myths that determine how we live out these larger myths: our choices, our fears, our dreams, our failures.

I have always been moved by Socrates' comment that the unexamined life is not worth living. It is only recently that I clearly understood that he said this shortly before he drank the hemlock. I had wanted his comment to be a guide for living; now it seems more a reflection designed to affirm the life he led. The fact that it ended as it ended may explain why so many people squirm at the thought of examining their lives. Maybe we're all afraid of what we will find. We hide things behind walls and pretend they cannot harm us since we have sequestered them so well. This is an illusion. They will come out and will have their way with us, one way or another, now and later.

Myths seem such forces to me, and while the examining of myths is difficult, sometimes harrowing, ignoring them is equally dangerous and has the added embarrassment of being stupid. So I vote with Socrates, hemlock and all, liking the integrity and autonomy afforded me by the examination. But such examination is not fun or easy, and it stands in sharp contrast to the more hedonistic models in vogue today: the avoidance of reflection or the cheap quick trick of emotive, sentimental, and superficial self-appraisal.

Myths shape everything. This is worrisome, of course. If you don't know your myths, you are busy shaping without knowing exactly what you're shaping. At the very least, this should evoke a certain nervousness. Folks end up saying things that they never meant to say. Conflict resolution efforts often seem this way to me. People of good faith, with good intentions, keep saying and doing things that seem to represent unexamined life at its best. Such people accept mythic assumptions and sanitize them for their purposes rather than scrutinizing and perhaps even transforming them. As a result, the mythic assumptions of the conflict become the mythic assumptions of the outcomes, and all parties fail to imagine that alternate mythic images might serve them better. Einstein once said that imagination is more important than knowledge. Conflict resolution often seems more intent on knowledge than on imagination, more on facticity than wisdom.

This is inherently contradictory, since the generation of options is a central task of negotiation. Such option generation seems to me the most creative and fun part of conflict resolution. If facticity and the sustaining of central myths are placed as constraints on this task, the options will be narrow and unimaginative and will further perpetuate the problems that gave rise to the conflict. This seems difficult to confront. When I have seen efforts made to do so, they are often dismissed as trivial. When I have tried to do so myself with very accomplished negotiators, I sense an inner conflict in such persons. They seem to say, "Yes, you are right, but there is no solution to this quandary, and besides, it scares me and I don't want to look at it or think about it, even a little. Please go away!"

This is not comforting to me. It also creates waves of self-doubt. It makes me more careful in my reflections. It has not, however, silenced the inner voice that tells me that conflict resolution has not yet arrived at the soul of the matter. What is perhaps more ominous is the sense that there is no intention of ever getting there. Often people merely fine-tune the superficial layers of a problem, avoiding the deeper issues implicit in conflict resolution. Myth is a central issue in this regard. It is an American myth that if it works for you it must not be broke, and if it ain't broke, you shouldn't fix it. Imagining airplanes or electricity did not emerge from this myth.

The myths of our past take us to the heart of any matter. The myths of our future are the outpourings of imagination. Both are integral to the tough task of creating desired outcomes when we're confronted with a conflict. Neither seem to me to be adequately acknowledged in current explorations of conflict resolution. Intuitively, one or another negotiator may "cheat" and use these gifts at a given moment. This does not make the negotiators credible, but rather examples of deviance. This is not enough for me.

Revealing the Shadow Side

My years of working in conflict resolution have actually deepened my understanding of our attachment to dominance power. Carl Jung (1958) created a road map for this understanding; it took life experiences to help me actually walk the path he describes so well. Jung posited that to achieve comprehensive self-knowledge one must look at both that which we view as our "goodness" and that which we view as our "badness" (Jung, 1963). He coined the word shadow in referring to the latter, the traits we store in the unconscious because we have learned that they are wrong. It is the shadow side that acts on and then defends our sense of entitlement, claiming the right to control others, stripping them of their autonomy and freedoms. Jung rightly noted that the shadow, unrevealed, was a moral problem.

The shadow contains those qualities we know can bring us shame, make us feel weak or petty, reveal the evil in our hearts. We deny this evil. It persists, manifesting in indirect ways. Doggedly, we insist that it is nonexistent. In times of conflict, this insistence inflates, and the shadow can determine our behaviors and their outcomes. When in conflict I want to sketch a picture of the other as evil, myself as virtuous, in the "right."

This foray into reflections on the shadow side is important. Some persons set uneven tables because their shadow side sustains inequities as a means of sustaining dominance power. Persons who reveal the unevenness of a table can therefore activate this shadow side, and evoke strong, sometimes harmful responses. Denial of the shadow and denial of a fixation on dominance power are often commingled unconsciously. Hence, the intent to reveal the uneven table concurrently can reveal the shadow side of those who set such tables. Such revelations, unsought and unwelcome, can create some harrowing events for those doing the revealing.

This sounds a bit ominous, and sometimes it truly is. While I alluded to this in the first edition of this book, I now give this process more focused attention. As I have gone about the United States teaching people about uneven tables, I have become increasingly motivated to do so. While many, indeed most persons find the discussions that reveal uneven tables to be quite liberating and clarifying, in nearly every audience there is one person (sometimes three or four) for whom acknowledgement of the uneven table evokes intense, protective, angry, even retaliatory responses. Inevitably I find myself facing the shadow of another.

This is important to note because such encounters are often destructive and cruel. They have a strong flavor of righteousness about them, and have often led to descriptions of me in terms incongruent with my behaviors and traits. It has taken me several years to understand that the pattern of projection and blaming discussed later in this book is particularly virulent when the projection involves another's shadow. I note this only to observe that perhaps no deterrent to honestly abandoning dominance power is as great as the projection of one's shadow onto another. The next step becomes "justifiable" violence against this other.

While I was writing the first edition to this book, my older brother Bob, who is a scripture scholar, was writing a book that was also on conflict (Beck, 1996). His involved the biblical Gospel of Mark and traced the roots of nonviolence expressed there, as well as the relationship of those roots to the work of Mohandas Gandhi, Martin Luther King Jr., and those who follow their approaches to nonviolence. He posited that the antithesis to their worldview was expressed in Louis L'Amour's work, fictional stories about men who engage in "justifiable" violence, that is, men who are permitted to be violent because they have "right" on their side, are retaliating to prevail over evil. When I project my own evil, my shadow, on to others, using L'Amour's rationale, I not only get to call them evil; I also get to do them harm.

Training others in conflict resolution has taught me the tight hold L'Amour's work has on our imaginations, and how deeply this is linked to our convictions about dominance power. It has also sensitized me to the cultural pattern of projection of the shadow. If I can declare myself to be in the right, know I should prevail, and then find myself opposed, then the person who opposes me is obviously evil (because I clearly am not) and can be destroyed without guilt. Consequently I prevail, as I should, and have power over the others who, benighted, do not have the same level of goodness and wisdom that guides me.

This even looks sort of foolish when written out so candidly. Yet it is a central dynamic in the U.S. culture. Now, should someone enter the dialogue challenging these destructive patterns of denial of the shadow, shadow projection, and attachment to dominance power, then that person of course is very evil, and very deserving of destructive retaliation: why colonists kill the rebellious natives. No mystery here, but a template for a culture's patterns of violence and hatred.

An obvious alternative is confrontation with one's own shadow. Indeed I am increasingly convinced that my skills as a negotiator are directly related to the depth of both self-revelation and integration of my shadow. This of course is not good news for those deeply attached to denial and projection of the shadow. I empathize a bit, but note that I did not invent this reality; I merely discovered it experientially. If my life experiences are any indicator, this is a pretty important discovery.

Zweig and Wolf wrote *Romancing the Shadow: Illuminating the Dark Side of the Soul* in 1997. In it, they posit that we can elect to form a relationship with this shadow side of ourselves, hence building a more conscious relationship with the contents of the unconscious. Dream analysis is an example of such work. In creating this relationship, they note, we free ourselves from blaming others and liberate the creative energy trapped in the unconscious. We also begin to discover that power over others, often used to suppress the shadow, is a fairly unimaginative activity, even a boring one. In freeing ourselves, we support the freedoms of others.

Integrating our shadow side is yet another way of releasing the deep insecurity that drives the need to control others. I am not likely to imagine alternatives to dominance power without a conscious effort to reveal my shadow side, to watch it at work, and to elect to restrain its hankering for "justifiable" violence.

Johnson and Ruhl (1999) take this exploration a step further, unveiling the links we forge between our projections and our conflicts. Their intent is to discuss contentment, and thus they identify projection primarily as a deterrent to such contentment. They note that projection involves "attaching an aspect of your inner life onto someone or something on the outside" (p. 36). In essence, my inner conflict, projected, becomes an inappropriately externalized conflict. It also results in surrendering my moral agency to another. The other now possesses my evil and I no longer can influence the impact of this evil: "you endow other people and things with the power to make you blissful or miserable" (p. 36).

Johnson and Ruhl believe we can learn to recognize when projection is at work: our response typically will be "(1) emotional, (2) compulsive, and (3) out of proportion to the reality of the situation" (p. 42). These indicators provide a practical guide to both self-assessment and conflict analysis. Learning both the clues to my projection of my shadow and the shadow projection embedded in conflicts I confront can give me access to substantive alternatives to justifiable violence.

One last observation of Johnson and Ruhl rounds out this discussion of imagining alternatives. They observe that not only individuals but also whole groups and societies engage in shadow projection, positing that this is the basis for "cultural, racial, and religious prejudices and conflicts." They note that "all scapegoating is due to projection" (pp. 46–47). These insights into shadow projection can provide powerful tools in understanding the conflicts that emerge at uneven tables, and the behaviors that express these conflicts. Shadows count.

7

Illusions We Live By

While respect for mystery and revealing the shadow can help us find those aspects of ourselves that distort our efforts at conflict resolution, metaphors and myths can be used to sustain illusions that keep us from ultimate, substantive realities. They contain and sustain our distortions, our misconceptions, our fears, our vanities, our self-preoccupations. They keep us at the brink of continual conflict, because the nasty voice of reality seems always lurking, ready to challenge and destroy our illusions. Illusions need a lot of protecting. Myths and metaphors help. They are like fortress walls or first lines of defense. The use of a war metaphor is appropriate here, because an illusion is always a self-construction that is not congruent with reality. It must, therefore, be sustained by avoiding the intrusion of reality, which reveals the incongruence. If the illusion is important to me, I am willing to fight off reality to sustain the illusion. This is a central human conflict, a familiar face of the human condition. It is often our preferred approach to concealing our shadow side.

Illusions are also comforting. They free us from uncertainty, ambiguity, mystery. They tell us that despite our nervous apprehension that everything is always changing, always in motion, here at least, in our little illusion, we have stability, sameness, certainty. This situation feels better than the challenge of living with ambiguity, uncertainty, change. But illusions are not only a source of comfort; they are also a trap. To keep them intact, we must freeze the flow of life, get out of the river and set up a camp on the shore, put down roots, become fixed and stable. Taking this safe course keeps us warm at night, but it can kill our imagination. It puts fetters on our images of human possibilities.

A larger question is lurking here, of course. What is stable? We are a nation in transition on this question. We have all, at some level of our hearts and souls, tried to make peace with questions of transcendence: is there more than what I can sense, is there some larger force than myself and my peers, is the larger power positive or negative, controlling or liberating, or is the question stupid to start with? The answers to these questions are, of course, the rich soil of metaphor, myth, and illusion. What we frame as answers will tell us a great deal about the metaphors we embrace, the myths we reproduce in our lives, and thus the illusions we create and sustain. And these things are ultimately the basis for all of our conflicts.

We seem reluctant to admit this. We tend in our culture to reduce the profound roots of conflict to simple power plays. But people die and are passionate in war because of differences. It doesn't require brilliance to note that most wars stem from differences based on definitions of god and religion. Amusingly, because we in America know we're right about our definitions of god and religion, we don't admit that this is the basis for our claim. It all depends, of course, on what you view as god and religion. Science can be a god, personal freedom a religion; consumerism can be a god, material greed a religion; control can be a god, democracy a religion. Here our imaginations have been fairly productive. We have an extensive array of options if we are out shopping for gods or for religions. And these creations, so deeply cherished, are things we'll die for if need be. Questioning all this is called treason. It might equally be called heresy. As confining illusions go, this is paradigmatic.

Tinkering on the Surface

Ignoring the importance of metaphors, myths, and illusions can lead to some pretty superficial activity, devoid of imagination or innovative thought. Boundaries on any endeavor constrict and confine, limiting creative output. Hence, one is left with a sense of tinkering with the surface phenomena, of trying to move chess pieces on a board without acknowledging the presence of tectonic plates beneath them. One good shift of the tectonic plates and the whole chessboard and all the pieces disappear. The deeper truths explain more, despite the increase in mystery and ambiguity. The struggle to go beyond tinkering is worth the effort, even if the discomfort level increases.

I imagine sometimes that human discourse occurs on one hundred levels. The choice of one hundred is arbitrary, used only to connote multiplicity. I also imagine sometimes that human discourse is like a large, hundred-spoke wheel. The choice of one hundred is again arbitrary. In each image, I am trying to capture my sense that one can acknowledge complexity. In the levels image, I honor depth and in the wheel image I honor scope. Both seem functional to me. Merged, they become a long spiral. Indeed, that is one of my images of myself, a long spiral. And when I have genuine human exchange with a loved and valued other, I experience this a bit like a DNA molecule: two interacting and interfaced spirals.

Whenever discourse seems disjointed to me, it is because some levels are unknown, withheld, denied, forbidden access, or simply not yet a part of awareness and consciousness. Some spokes of the wheel evoke the same images. Hence, discourse with others is marked by the depth and scope of their self-awareness and my self-awareness. This has motivated me to steadily increase my self-awareness, because I am curious and seem unwilling to miss anything. It has also been my experience that some people can help me discover my levels and spokes by manifesting theirs as a mirror, or reflecting their sense of mine back to me. I like this exchange, indeed I am deeply enthused by it. I have noticed, however, that it seems dependent on my willingness to see. When I resist seeing, it is usually because I have an illusion I'm protecting, a myth I have failed to explore, a metaphor that enslaves me, or a shadow aspect of myself I am denying. I also notice that if I don't go beyond these constraints, I miss out on a lot of life, creativity, joy, pleasure, fun, and fulfillment. Unfortunately, to go beyond my constraints, I have to slog my way through a swampland of fear, pride, and stubbornness to overcome my resistance to new experiences. I don't always measure up to the challenge. When I do, I am joyful; when I don't, I am diminished. This helps keep me slogging. The opposite of slogging, for me, is tinkering on the surface.

One can transform deterrents, if one wishes to do so. Reframing such deterrents can actually become fairly entertaining. Rather than fear looking at my illusions, I am more and more inclined to fear an unlived and unexamined life, a depletion and constriction, a failure to become. Rather than protecting my vanity by denying unpleasant distortions and misconceptions, I am developing a sizable vanity about living on the edge, being willing to grapple with life, shadows, illusions and all, being willing to acknowledge my mistakes and take responsibility for both their consequences and the need to correct them, being courageous enough to live my own truth. Rather than stubbornly defending my own self-will, I am learning to become stubborn about fidelity to the possible, the imaginable, the new vision, and equally to the acceptability of the human condition in all its poverty and limitation. These lessons have proven liberating, albeit challenging.

Which is to say, of course, that I am not interested in furthering the effort to tinker on the surface. It seems cowardly to me now, as well as intellectually foolish. Some days it even seems dangerous and tragic. I am not naïve, however, about how many people like to live where I live, and I am not willing to pretend they are there if they are not. This makes me irritating sometimes, I think. Still, better a little irritation than a war. It took me more than fifty years to figure out that it is better to experience a little anxiety and evoke a little irritation than it is to tinker on the surface. I don't even hang out with tinkerers anymore. I figure with so many people eager to sustain the status quo, they don't need my help with the effort. Besides, we nontinkerers need one another desperately. I find them, and I bond. I cherish them.

Explorations of conflict that tinker on the surface are thus less-than-satisfying experiences for me. They seem to invite confinement intellectually, emotionally, morally, spiritually—humanly. Saying this can also render me irritating. Nonetheless, I am committed to moving beyond tinkering on the surface. The monsters and demons lurking on the other levels, the scary visions on the other spokes need some unveiling. Only then will we move toward deeply imaginative creations that address the conflicts implicit in the human condition. We may even discover the demons are angels in disguise, the creativity of our shadow side described by Jung.

Wider and Deeper Visions of Reality

Sometimes people think that if you seek wider and deeper visions, you are a better person. I don't think so. I think most people learn to seek wider and deeper visions of reality because they notice that they are not all that great, and that they are clearly not better than anyone else. They start noticing that wider and deeper visions may be their best option for coping with their limitations. They notice that having many people solving a problem at least leads to a wider array of options for consideration and often leads to a better solution. They also notice that if lots of people help create the solution, they are more likely to embrace the solution, and implementation goes more smoothly. Finally, they like not being alone in their humanness. They like being part of a community of limited humans slogging out the possible solution they can find to a demanding dilemma. In that sense, wider and deeper vision enhances my outcomes.

Some other dimensions to seeking a wider and deeper solution, however, are more troublesome. Some people think that if they do so they themselves are actually better. This is pretty sneaky thinking. It can veil a goofy kind of vanity that deters creativity and constricts the outcome to the vision of the one vain person. If such persons are vain, they are also probably fearful that their idea won't prevail, and so fear gets mixed in. They then need to prevail to assuage their fears and to nourish their vanity. We all have these drifts on occasion, but if it is the prevailing drift, wider and deeper vision may not ultimately improve our outcomes.

Some people also like someone else to have wider and deeper visions for them, and so they then award all responsibility to these people. They forego self-responsibility and create unwise dependencies on others. They also create a climate where other people can get caught in the vanity trap described above. People who forego responsibility eventually don't like something these others do and try to reclaim their rights. This can really upset those who have gotten accustomed to being in charge. So this too can be a way that wider and deeper visions may not create desired outcomes.

As noted earlier, the effort to move toward wider and deeper visions eventually elicits the need to reveal one's personal shadow side. Now the visions themselves may be quite an attractive option, but slogging through the muck of one's shadow may appear excessive. After all, years were spent burying these "negative" traits, and more poignantly, convincing others that the traits belonged to some arbitrarily chosen "other" who is actually the problem. Shadow work is painful and time-consuming, so sometimes people decide that wider and deeper visions are just too demanding.

Such persons may just find wider and deeper visions too demanding. They have an array of options. They may choose to avoid the whole messy thing. They may be polite and appear to be going along with the wider and deeper agenda, but inside they have checked out of the room. They may mention all of the deficiencies of wider and deeper, over and over again, or they may go silent, passive, unreachable, and scare or intimidate others. They may try to project all the obstacles to wider and deeper, all the murky shadow content, onto others. They may try to make wider and deeper visions simple, easy—a variant on tinkering on the surface. They may thus create facile solutions to complex problems and insist that they have done so in a nice wide and deep way. In these ways also, wider and deeper may not bring forth desired outcomes.

Nonetheless, despite these risks, I opt for wider and deeper visions. This approach is imperfect, but it is at least honest in its imperfections. It gives me a chance to affirm my own struggling humanity, and it gives me a chance to affirm the struggling humanity of others. I am uncertain if the outcomes are better; there is no real way of honestly testing this. I am certain that it is a better human outcome, and since conflict is first a human thing, what fits and benefits the humans seems germane.

8

Beyond Appearances

I'm a little worried now that you think I took a wrong turn and got lost in philosophical musings that fail to get you closer to your goal of figuring out what I have to say about uneven tables. There is a method to my madness, however. We're nearing the end of Part One of this book. All along, I've been trying to warn you about the seduction of easy solutions, facile answers, and shallow compromises. As we proceed further, the seduction will become more palpable.

This is why I have described my assumptions. They do not support the easy, facile, or shallow outcome, and if you choose it, I have at least been clear. You may elect to tinker on the surface of conflict, deny and project your shadow side, sustain and protect your illusions, and leave your myths and metaphors unexamined. That is your choice. It is not my message. I am now practicing another way of being at an uneven table: drawing a line in the sand without cruelty.

Getting By and Getting Even

Most of us work to "get by" when confronted with conflict. The popularized version of this in the United States is captured in the colloquial expression of "getting even." When we experience unevenness, the "getting by" recommended is to "get even." We like to think, when we try to "get even," that we are addressing substantive values of justice, fair play, balance, and equality. We like to think that "getting even" reflects the fundamental tenets of the belief systems and the economic, political, and social structures we cherish.

Getting even, however, is awash in distortion. It suggests vengeance and deception—behaviors that inevitably diminish a person. More subtle, however, is the fantasy that it works. When we experience unevenness and try to "get even," we usually tell ourselves that we only want what is our "due" and that those who have "more than their due" should give up some for us. The persons with "more," of course, believe that this is their due and will not give it up. If we succeed in taking our "due" from them, they will feel that this is an injustice, and turn, like us, and try to get even. This is at best an entitlement exchange.

It does not require extraordinary insight to see that this model is somewhat flawed. Despite this, it persists as a popular problem-solving device. Secretly, we harbor the hope that once we "get even," everything will be all right, and life will manifest a gracious balance. Instead, we find ourselves dealing with people trying to "get even" with us for having gotten even with them. There is a boring repetitiveness in all of this, a circular futility. When the process involves powerful personal relationships, or toxic substances in our water supply, or nuclear weapons, it goes well beyond simple futility and boredom.

All of which is to say that you can turn fainthearted now, looking back longingly to the days when you knew exactly what to do with unevenness, or you can tackle the challenge. It is of course the stuff of evolution. If you consent to at least temporarily suspend the seduction to "get even," the demands of expanding your vision are worth pondering. Half measures have their own destructive outcomes and create their own tragic consequences.

The Dangers of a Partial Reframe

One of the most challenging aspects of understanding uneven tables is the fact that it is easier to recognize when you are at one as the participant viewed as less than equal than it is to recognize when you are at one as the person who is advantaged in some way. As much as I may find uneven tables disturbing when I am disadvantaged, this awareness does not ensure that I will realize when others feel disadvantaged. In some cases, it may even make me less aware. I may be so taken with the "measuring" of my disadvantage, or so frustrated with the impact of my disadvantage on outcomes, that I may fail to see my advantages. This worsens the impact of the uneven table.

A particularly virulent strain of this virus involves attachment to disadvantage. I may have found some quite comforting secondary gains in being disadvantaged, or I may like the fact that someone else has to take all the risks and has all the responsibility. I may have been taught that I didn't deserve advantages, and harbor guilts that make me subvert my efforts to seek and acquire opportunities. I may have become attached to suffering as an explanation for life, a way to avoid the challenge of growth and change. All these can be ways of embracing, often unconsciously, a partial reframe. In the end, they are as dangerous as the unethical wielding of dominance power for destructive ends.

It is equally dangerous to embrace predigested and unexamined social constructions that predict unevenness: sexism, racism, ageism, anti-intellectualism, and other equally attractive "isms." This is the threat of political correctness as unreflective oversimplification. We then hope that we need not examine our own beliefs, values, attitudes, and behaviors, but merely "plug in" the proper view and emerge egalitarian. We also hope to elude our emotions, thinking that thinking is the critical factor. Most of us can think some pretty lovely thoughts, and this assures nothing in behavior and attitudes. Emotions endure, no matter how cleverly we think we have costumed them. Shadows lurk, and influence.

The ability to clearly recognize unevenness in its many guises is simply not that simple. Most of us can conjure a list where we feel disadvantaged. We can also conjure a list where we think we can anticipate that others might feel disadvantaged. The greater challenge is to find our own blindnesses, where we are advantaged and fail to recognize it, where our disadvantage can serve as an advantage, where someone else we believe to be advantaged is actually disadvantaged.

This is another danger of the partial reframe. We convince ourselves that we have exhausted the opportunities for insight into the threats of unevenness. We probably can never do that, given the complexity and mystery of the human heart and soul. My impeccable logic about what and how others should feel rarely determines what and how they feel.

We would like to imagine that there are a predictable set of knowables that can provide a predictive guide to current sources of unevenness. We would like to imagine that we can memorize this list and then magically free ourselves from the threat of unevenness. We like to imagine that we can exhaust human mystery. Amusingly, if others imply that they have exhausted our mystery, we may prove a bit less simplistic in our appraisal.

I don't think we can exhaust human mystery. I've been amazed at how difficult I find it to really know myself in all my mystery, and I think I'm motivated, engaged, and competent. I'm always turning up a new firefly of creativity in the backyard moonlight, or another slug of shadow imperfection under a rock. If I have this much trouble grasping my own mystery, where I have fairly consistent access to the database, how much more difficult to exhaust the mystery of another person, where the access is less consistent. Mystery just is. It is of course one of life's adventures that mystery cannot be exhausted.

I have written this book with the assumption that mystery just is, and that therefore it makes more sense to develop the skills I need to negotiate at an uneven table than it does to try to force all tables to become even, or to feed the illusion that they can become even. I don't think they can, either in some large detached-observer sense or in the minute-to-minute process sense. If I can't have my fantasy, it makes sense to me to figure out what to do with what I have in its stead.

The fact is, it is impossible to elude the uneven table. Somewhere, everyone gets to sit at one. When the unevenness is dramatic, we know it clearly. More often, however, we sense it intuitively or instinctively. We know things aren't quite fair, that something lopsided is happening and we are part of it. If we're at the table to resolve a conflict, this lopsidedness portends a failure to resolve the conflict, and we begin to wonder exactly why we're at the table and what we can do about the situation.

If we acknowledge these realities, we are able to shift our focus from the illusion that we can, should, or have set an even table to the recognition that no table is even, and that the skills needed to meet the challenge of unevenness are a better use of human creativity. As much as I try to imagine all tables becoming even, the image just never conjures clearly. But if I concede that the uneven table is a given, my options expand.

Finding a way to be at an uneven table offers many benefits. If I feel forced to be at this table, or silenced, or discounted, or if I feel somehow that I am being required to forgo the opportunity to "have voice," the idea of alternatives attracts me. It gets me to every table I might want to be at, gives me an opportunity to make a difference. I can always leave if I choose to do so.

If I am the advantaged person in such a negotiation, the challenge is often more subtle for me, but no less persuasive. I claim to have come to the table to resolve a conflict. If my advantage furthers the conflict, I need to realize that it is not in my self-interest to further the conflict by denying my advantage. Conversely, I may have to face the somewhat embarrassing fact that I am there not to resolve the conflict but to "win." This challenge is sneakier than it looks.

A Story

When I was a dean of a school of nursing, an opportunity presented itself to create a health care clinic in a part of an urban inner city where virtually no health care was available. I was deeply troubled by the lack of health services for people without resources, and I believed that responding to this opportunity was congruent with the school's mission and the values and commitments of nursing. I pursued the opportunity.

This involved a complex set of negotiations with a state funding agency, several city agencies, the school and university communities, and most important, the neighborhood residents. I slogged my way through a morass of politically sensitive negotiations and eventually reached the final negotiation, the one with representatives of the neighborhood. I think I wanted a thank-you note. I had taken a number of political risks getting to this final table.

The neighborhood representatives explained to me that the only viable clinic was one they would eventually control. I agreed. They explained that it should be created with this assumption. I agreed. They noted that the way that they would set up a clinic and run it, and the way that I, my school, my university, the city agencies, or the state would set up a clinic differed. I panicked. I was not invested in creating something that a whole choir of political voices had assumed was going one way, and the residents might very likely take along a completely different path. It could be a path all the other parties didn't like.

I had managed to give lip service to community control of health care most of my career. I believed that much health care was ethnically inappropriate, that we had devised health care models responsive to the beliefs and values of Americans of European ancestry but insensitive to Americans of just about every other culture of origin. I thought these things should change. Yet, when confronted by the practical costs of those beliefs, I discovered how easy it was for me to become cowardly.

I knew I had taken many risks to get to this point in the negotiations. I knew that I had an advantage; after all, I was the dean. I could hear this voice in my head screaming for safety, wanting to sustain my control of the clinic so I would not have all the forces of the political choir raging at me for failing to create the clinic that fit their imaginings. I knew the residents wanted one that fit their needs, and that they had historically been disadvantaged health care consumers because care simply didn't fit. They wanted a clinic that was truly different, one responsive to their world.

The ensuing inner battle I had with myself was a deeply personal learning experience. I was embarrassed, tripping over my own secret desire to retain control of the clinic for my own safety and vanity. Once deeper and wider thinking came to my rescue, I participated in an ongoing series of careful negotiations that in the end ensured community control. My contribution was not one of control, but of serving as monitor, identifying those initiatives that could destroy the potential of the clinic for good should it offend too many political forces too deeply. I was not the controlling advantaged person, but a resource to the community, a bridge between the community and the political choir. They, in turn, honored my requests for attention to my concerns.

In the end, I believe the gains from this demanding learning experience so overshadow the petty possibilities of controlling a clinic that I blush in retrospect. The willingness of the community representatives to educate me, confront me, be patient with me while I struggled, teach me, forgive me, comfort me, attend to my safety, and thank me seems enormous beside the small comfort of an illusion of control. Retrospectively, the contrast seems stark. One does not discover the limits of the illusion of control until one lets go of the illusion and tries alternatives. In this case, had I failed to face the seduction of my own advantage, many people who should have had health care would have lost the opportunity. Blindness had implications.

This clinic lesson unveiled some other important issues for me about evolutionary change. The demographic distribution of ethnic groups in the United States is changing and will continue to change. Being European American when I was a child was operationally "normative." Ozzie and Harriet were not Hispanic, and the father that knew best was not African American. Each day, these norms shift. What was once an advantage ceases to be so as these changes progress, no matter how much some people might long for the past. In addition, what was once a disadvantage ceases to be so. This is true not only of ethnicity, but also of gender, age, health status, sexual preference, and a variety of other ways that people differ. When an imbalance occurs, eventually the species struggles back to balance.

Hence, a clear understanding of where unevenness is assumed to exist is important not only for ascertaining where there might be an uneven table, but also for ascertaining where there might be an inappropriate assumption of one. This latter case creates another type of uneven table. All types are germane. It seems useful to list here some of the current categories used to predict privilege, since they are by now lurking in your mind. The following list is not exhaustive but gives some broad general categories. This may prove comforting to you if you're a reader who just knows that one of these groups has been driving you to distraction with its irritating privileges.

Assumptions About Privilege

Today, in the United States, many people assume the following to be true with respect to privilege:

- European American persons are more privileged than persons from other cultures.

- Wealthy persons are more privileged than indigent persons.

- Persons who are men are more privileged than persons who are women.

- Professional persons are more privileged than persons who are laborers.

- Persons in management positions are more privileged than persons in employee positions.

- Able-bodied persons are more privileged than persons who are physically challenged.

- Healthy persons are more privileged than persons who are ill.

- Strong persons are more privileged than weak persons.

- Persons who present themselves as rational are more privileged than persons who present themselves as emotional.

This list guides a great deal of public discourse. It currently evokes a good deal of political rhetoric, legislative debate, media attention, and personal interaction. We attend to these issues, sometimes defensively or defiantly, sometimes guiltily or self-righteously, sometimes with anxious denial and distancing.

I'm kind of hoping by now you may have noticed that there is a value assumption in the list. The value assumption is that control predicts privilege; that power and agency (and their legal tender—money) are the indicators of advantage. We operationalize this assumption daily and reinforce it repeatedly, until the unreflective person begins to assume that it is reality. Anyone who has watched a strong, rational, wealthy, healthy, and able-bodied European American man who is a professional manager hope for a hug from his child and not receive it knows intuitively that there is something missing from this list.

An Exercise

Find or purchase a newsmagazine. Start from the front and review each article or item. Reflect on each a while. Then determine if the unstated focus of the article is dominance power. Make two lists: articles where you decide the focus is dominance power and those where it is not. Count the lists and compare the two numbers.

Now take the lists and revisit those articles where you decided the focus was not dominance power. Briefly record what you think the focus was. Review this list. The task now becomes more subtle. If not power, what? Fame, success, money, popularity, sex? Or their opposites: shame, deprivation, defeat, poverty, tragedy, isolation, failure, disaster? Reread the articles. Why are these themes important to us? How many are actually the prerequisites or the rewards for dominance power? How many focus on the indicators of the cost of its absence?

Now that you have located all the instances of dominance power, its incentives and its threats, what's left in the news?

The reality is that privilege and advantage have many measures. Everyone is underprivileged and disadvantaged in some way. It is important to get accustomed to this idea early on, since habits of the mind are hard to break and can blind and enslave the best of us. Imagining the ways we perceive others to be privileged or underprivileged can be a useful exercise. Control itself can be a disadvantage. It can prevent us from experiencing other meaningful dimensions of what it means to be human. It can require us to avoid making mistakes at any cost to sustain that control. It can demand that we take responsibility for any number of persons who choose not to be responsible for themselves. It can take seven years off of our life expectancy.

It is equally important to acknowledge that privilege on some measures does exist, that in some dimensions we are either not all created exactly equal or deterred in some way from exercising an intrinsic equality. In some cases, the deterrent is socially structured inequity. Thus, pursuing equity despite an entire society full of deterrents can be difficult at best. These deterrents are real, and the discounting of such deterrents by those not confronting them adds insult to injury. It also demonstrates that our national commitments to justice are in some way not yet honored, that democracy does not yet prevail.

Balance in facing these realities is a difficult challenge. People who are societally disadvantaged can avoid self-responsibility and play out a victim role, rebel, or withdraw from the efforts at justice. People who are societally advantaged can abuse the privilege along a continuum from modestly innocuous to seriously harmful injustices; they can sustain the injustices by denial and avoidance. These dynamics need to be acknowledged.

Victims and victimizers need one another. Where you have one, you must have the other. If you scratch the surface of this dynamic, you will also find its obverse, where the victim inevitably becomes a victimizer in some fashion, and the victimizer thus becomes a victim. For this reason alone, understanding unevenness is meritorious, despite the challenge. Since you've read this far, I'm banking on your being one of the folks who are at least curious if there is some other way to attend to all this than the popularized version: keeping the old frames on reality alive and well.

This book focuses on the skills needed to sit at a table where you believe you or others are problematically participating with less privilege than others. It offers an alternative to acquiring, sustaining, or imposing victim behavior. It's hard to be a victimizer if no one volunteers to be the victim. Being victimized day to day is bad enough. If you negotiate at a table on your own behalf, purportedly in a spirit of self-interest, you need skills beyond those of the victim. To do so, you must deliberately elect to move beyond the traditional behaviors manifested by people at an uneven table. The next section of this book will give you a chance to better familiarize yourself with those behaviors.

Before we turn to that, however, I want to commend you for reading this first part of the book. Some people probably skipped it. These sloths will try to tell you at a cocktail party someday that they read this book. This is a test to see if they were as honest as you are about really reading the whole book.

I'm going to tell you a story. It actually doesn't have anything to do with this book, but that makes this even better. Then, when you meet people who claim they've read the book, you can say to them enthusiastically, "Didn't you love the story about the baseball hat?" or "My favorite was the story about the family game of football; wasn't the part about halftime great!" Then watch closely. If they give you a blank, anxious, or furtive look, you can feel self-righteous for having read the whole book, including Part One, which has some pretty demanding chunks in it.

Like many parents, I like to tell stories about my kids. Here's the story.

A Story

When my kids were younger, their father and I would take them to a park to play. My younger daughter wanted one thing more than anything else for her third birthday, a baseball cap. We had honored her request and she wore it at all times, including to bed. It was a sacred totem. So she was of course wearing it one weekend when we went to a local park.

We brought along a football and decided we would play a little touch football. The teams were drawn: Dad and Patty against Mom and Becky. Patty was four years older than Becky. (Mom knew this was something of an uneven table, or playing field: maybe this is about the book after all!) It was less of an issue for Becky, who understood the purpose of play better than any of us.

First we negotiated the fact that Becky was the only one with a proper hat. Becky was reluctant to play with three dolts who had failed to bring the proper equipment. We pointed out that she had a baseball hat, not a football helmet. She pointed out that this fine distinction was irrelevant. She alone had come adequately prepared to engage in serious sport.

We then set up for our first play. Becky and I had possession, and I told her I would hand off to her. I told her some numbers I would say, and then when I got to a specific number, I would hand her the ball. She was then to run as fast as she could toward an indicated tree, making a glorious touchdown for the underdogs. I would hold off Dad and Patty while she ran like a deer.

We set up and I said the numbers, handed the ball to Becky, and began trying to keep Patty and Dad from her. She made it to the tree, while the three dolts without proper equipment stood dumbfounded. After I had handed Becky the ball, she carefully set it down, put her hand on her head to keep the baseball cap from blowing off, and ran for the tree. I had failed to mention that she was to take the ball with her.

While the three dolts stood in the middle of the football field explaining the fine details of the sport to Becky, she then announced that it was half-time and it was time for the parade. She lined up the more confused participants in the experience, and we all began marching up and down the football field making amazing music and stunning the crowds with our rendition of several children's songs.

What is of worth and value is in the eye of the beholder. Sometimes it is best found in the mind and heart of a child.

Part Two

Traditional Approaches to an Uneven Table

9

Manipulation as Tradition

There are two essential elements in solving a problem. Many people only want to address the second one: identifying solutions and selecting the best among them for implementation. The first element, often more challenging, is to clearly name, understand, and comprehend the full nature of a problem. I myself have often tried to skip this aspect of problem solving. I would rather fold clean laundry than sort dirty stuff scooting down the clothes chute.

Over time, I have become convinced that my solutions are as good as the care with which I endure stage one. If I don't fully understand a problem, I tend to come up with too few options or even get lost generating solutions to some unrelated albeit interesting other problem. These errors have become so embarrassing to me that I am now fairly adamant about grasping problems before I try to implement solutions.

Sometimes people tell me that they think I am being "negative," stubbornly insisting on naming and describing problems before I try to solve them. They tell me that no one else wants to do this, so what is "my problem"? They assure me that going through the first stage of problem solving is a miserable business, depresses everyone, and makes people feel hopeless, so we should just skip it and get right to the fun stuff: implementing the solutions.

This has taught me that I am not the only one who has this problem with implementing solutions before I know the nature of the problem. It has also taught me at least part of the reason why we're all in search of clean dry laundry needing folding and so disturbed at the mound of sweaty shorts and smelly socks sitting in front of us. We tend to want to avoid the dimensions of ourselves that appear negative. We hope no one else is noticing and we try very hard not to notice ourselves. We fear that others may think this dirty-laundry side of our behavior is all that's there. We also harbor the fear that this may be true. And finally, we may or may not want to do anything about it. This discourages stage one problem solving. Shadows count.

All this comes as a warning. This part of this book is a bit like sorting dirty laundry. Just because you can get everything in the correct load, does not make the task any more pleasant. Still, it is the first step of the process, so I am proceeding despite this worrisome sense that you may not like confronting the dirty laundry of uneven tables.

Uneven tables are not something new, or unfamiliar. We all visit them. Sometimes we even feel trapped at them, with no choice but to sit there and try to figure out what to do with the situation. Usually one is not permitted to fall asleep, so, in various stages of wakefulness, we participate. Later, we may sense a vaguely unsettling rumble somewhere inside that assures us that this was not the most fun thing we've done this week.

Before we can constructively identify useful new ways of being at uneven tables, we need to better understand what is going on at those tables. Awareness of what doesn't work is an obvious reason for this. A more demanding reason, however, is the task of facing and owning what we're doing now, knowing how it looks and how it works, and deciding if we want to continue to use these behaviors. Otherwise, we will probably all just rush to new ways of being at an uneven table, pretend we understand the issues, and glue on a little new behavior whenever we have the impulse. We will probably then be engaging in a new version of the common denominator in most traditional ways of negotiating at an uneven table: manipulation.

An Exercise

Find your journal. If you have it sitting right there beside you, I want to take a few minutes to admire you. Now, before you read any further, write down what you think of when you hear the word manipulation.

Having done this, write down the five ways you most commonly use manipulation with others. We will revisit this list. If you couldn't think of any, write down, "I just can't seem to think of any!" We will revisit this too. If you could only come up with one or two ways, try to find other people who have read this book and find out how many they wrote down. Don't ask for the details, just the number.

Sustaining Manipulation Through Mental Manipulation

While the term manipulate can mean "to manage or utilize skillfully," it can also mean "to control or play upon by artful, unfair, or insidious means, especially to one's own advantage" and "to change by artful and unfair means so as to serve one's purpose." Manual dexterity—the subject of the first definition—connotes a strength. The latter two definitions connote deception for one's own gain. The word insidious is not a friendly word. The assumption in these definitions is one of injustice. The most traditional way of dealing with the injustice of an uneven table is to be unjust in response, but in an artful and insidious manner, with deceit.

Now this is a pretty strong assertion, of course, so it will need some substantiation. Most of us don't voluntarily acknowledge that we are pursuing agendas of deceit and injustice, even if the situation we find ourselves in invites this response. We have found some clever ways of explaining this type of deceit and injustice. We say "I was being politically astute," or "He was a control maniac; someone had to keep him in his place," or "She was trying to take over;

it was the only way to get her in line," or "I had to do what I had to do; the whole group was headed toward this stupid decision." These are forms of mental manipulation we engage in to avoid facing the fact that we engaged in the manipulation of others. We argue that the end justifies the means. We then claim the means we used weren't really all that awful, given the threat. In effect, we use mental manipulation to deny the fact that we were manipulative.

This little process can get pretty complex. Once one engages in a single denied manipulation, viewing manipulation as less than virtuous, one must then manipulate one's thinking. One does this first to avoid self-condemnation, and later to avoid criticism from others. This process can absorb a good deal of time and energy.

If you go to an uneven table, believe yourself to be unable to exercise overt power or self agency, believe the negotiation is about power as control over others, or want to exercise power and believe for one reason or another that you are not able to do so, the most readily available resource is manipulation. It is most effective when it is veiled so well that it can successfully be denied. This is not a particularly brilliant insight, nor is it unfamiliar. There is a whole library of books on how to use manipulation. Some admit that this is the dynamic; more often the admission is not made and the behavior is labeled something else, such as persuasion or cleverness. Most books of this nature are not titled How to Use Deceit and Injustice in Moments of Perceived Powerlessness.

Interestingly, some negotiation experts essentially recommend manipulation as the tool of choice for the negotiator. They may not use this term, but the behaviors described are essentially manipulative in nature. This may merely reflect the fact that negotiators often feel pretty powerless when a conflict becomes intense or personalized. It may also indicate a belief on the part of the negotiator that he or she is confined to dominant power as the only currency of interest in negotiations.

The first and hardest thing to face about traditional approaches to an uneven table is that they are manipulative and are designed to "get even" or achieve one's goals through deceit and injustice. What is more troublesome is that once manipulation is introduced as the dynamic of choice, it becomes acceptable behavior, and countermanipulation is introduced. This can escalate until it is difficult to determine whether the conflict is about a substantive issue or the deep feelings of revulsion we experience when subjected to unwelcome and harmful manipulations and countermanipulations. This explains, for instance, more conflict between men and women than almost anyone wants to admit.

The fact is, most of us don't like to feel manipulated. It offends and insults us. We may see through the manipulation and be indulgent about it, but it does not evoke admiration and trust. We feel diminished by it, and if we respond in kind, we are even more diminished. It does not evoke the best in us and often evokes the worst. Thus, while the process may be as common as horseflies on potato salad, this does not make it more attractive or desirable.

Shadow projection can further inform us about manipulation. If I am busy denying that I manipulate others, I can always project this behavior on to others. I can then claim that I had to be countermanipulative because "they" were. This is always reminiscent to me of children fighting on the playground . . . "he started it." Such an explanation, while useful in denying the shadow side of our conflicts, does not seem to image the best of what it means to be human.

We need to struggle a bit with this idea of manipulation. We have so normalized it in our culture that to describe it as troublesome has become quaint. We assume it is more like skin and bones: everybody comes with some. We accommodate it, and we counter it with little if any reflection. Since it is the most popular version of addressing unacknowledged unevenness in a negotiation, this normalization can leave us stuck with an ineffective, deceitful, and unjust model for addressing conflicts. It may help us understand why so few conflicts really get resolved, and why they often return to haunt us.

A Further Reframe on Dominance Power

Before we examine some of the many expressions of manipulation popularized in our culture, an alternate way of looking at dominant power may be useful. Because we use dominant power as a central currency, we can easily lose our way in the struggle to make sense of its presence in our lives. One reason for this is that we fail to discriminate about dominance power.

All of us eventually find situations in our lives where the exercise of dominance power makes sense to us. Corralling a two-year-old explorer about to test a busy street or a hot stove are easy exemplars. We would consider ourselves remiss if we failed to do so. The military exercise of dominant power that sought to end the travesty of genocide in Germany is another exemplar, this time at a global level. "Someone had to stop Hitler," we say, and we do not apologize.

The fact is, there are times when the exercise of dominant power is a moral good in our culture, and few if any would differ with the judgment of that good. Beyond these tidy exemplars, however, a sea of ambiguity lurks. Because we use dominant power to such excess, and have rendered it commonplace for virtually all problem-solving activities, we lose our sensitivity to the inappropriate use of dominant power. The line between saving your child from the busy street and beating your child for defiantly ignoring your wishes is hard for many adults to discover. The willingness to incarcerate Japanese Americans whose only "crime" was ethnicity while assaulting genocide in Germany reveals a certain national confusion.

It appears that we drift toward using dominant power both excessively and indiscriminately, with an absence of self-reflection. While there indeed may be times when this type of power is appropriate, they probably represent a small fraction of the times it is actually used. Many uses of dominant power are simply inappropriate. We exercise such control not only out of genuine need for safety or clarity of judgment but also out of fear, insecurity, vengeance, vanity, habit, self-will, boredom, and laziness. We have failed to honestly confront the many uses of dominant power that are simply unthinking habituation to cultural norms, reflecting a poverty of imagination to find alternatives. The proliferation of jails in our country is a useful exemplar of this drift.

This habituation leaves us not only using an inappropriate prob-lem-solving device much of the time, but also serves to perpetuate the lack of imagination. Then, because our outcomes are so non-sensical much of the time, we activate even more dominant power to protect ourselves from self-honesty, the courage to change, and the will to imagine a better solution. When dominant power is used where it is inappropriate, it is experienced by many people as a form of coercive overt manipulation. People feel that the assurance of freedom is abridged by the intrusion of a dominant power that determines their well-being in ways not acceptable to them. They feel their right to self-determination is diminished.

What this experience can reveal is that dominant power, when exercised inappropriately, is often perceived as a behavior that ini-tiates the manipulation cycle in others. People then respond with countermanipulation. This often confuses the person exercising dominant power if self-awareness is limited or absent. Thus, a potential way of looking at dominant power is that it is manipula-tive when exercised inappropriately, in an artful, deceitful, insidi-ous, or unjust manner. At such times, it often evokes a response of manipulation.

This insight is more important than it may seem. Many people who exercise dominant power assume it is a birthright and do so indiscriminately, in all manner of places, with all manner of out-comes. When they are responded to with manipulative maneuvers, it offends them. It is difficult for them to see that they started the cycle. Once a manipulation and a countermanipulation are initi-ated, the cycle often has an inexorable quality, escalating to absurd levels. The arms race is a useful example.

It is worth struggling with this idea for a while; it took me many years to finally grasp it, so I want to imagine that it is stretching you somewhat, too. If someone exercises dominant power where it is inappropriate to do so, he or she is essentially using deceit to say, "I have the right to control you," when this assertion is untrue or unjust. When we feel someone is trying to control us in ways that we think are inappropriate, we feel ourselves dealt with unjustly. If we are not permitted to question or challenge this experience, we also feel that we are being deceived, that our trust is diminished. Impaired trust does not lead to meaningful relating. We intuitively sense that we have been reduced from the status of person to the status of "thing," an object to exploit and use for someone else's purposes. We do not like this feeling.

This reframe on dominant power is one of many ways that the inability to discriminate rears its ugly head. Once we think a tool is useful, we like to use it everywhere, it seems. Discrimination is difficult. It calls for a reflectiveness that often seems to be unavailable in a culture accustomed to life in the fast lane. We compulsively keep doing what we're doing because we're not sure we want to see what we might see if we stopped and reflected. We also are afraid we wouldn't then know what to do instead.

We are a culture that tends to glorify the intellect, rational thinking, logic. Yet, where our emotions have gone awry and we're scared to face that fact, we waffle mentally and fail to make clear distinctions. This leads to sloppy problem solving. It may thus prove useful to imagine that dominant power is a worthwhile device that has a few valuable uses, emerging only rarely. All the other times we use it may indeed be invitations to a countermanipulation, and a conflict. The challenge then becomes not to deal with conflict, but to prevent it by trying to both discriminate clearly and find alternative approaches to dilemmas where the seduction of dominant power shows up inappropriately. This can actually prove to be a fascinating challenge to our creative thinking. It is also difficult. Here's a poem about that difficulty.

turn on the night light

i know the child who chases the moon,
butterfly net and jar in hand:
still not able, after all these years
to discriminate
the firefly from the fire.

   —pbk

A Couple of Caveats

Since the publication of the first edition of this book, I have had a few more years to hone my powers of discrimination. During that time, I traveled to most of the states in this country, usually to share the contents of this book, and also moved from the North to the South. Both have taught me a great deal.

The former taught me that there is a rich array of styles of manipulation throughout the United States, and for most of the members of oppressed groups, it is not just their strategy of choice. Often there is a deep conviction that it is the only choice. To abandon manipulation looks dangerous; to confront uneven tables even more so. The assumption is that such confrontation will evoke harrowing levels of interpersonal violence. This is understandably very frightening.

If this feared interpersonal violence does emerge, members of oppressed groups often want to retaliate, to return the interpersonal violence. Both the risk of interpersonal violence and fear of the impulse toward retaliation make it seem wise to cling to manipulative behaviors.

This has drawn me to a reflective revisit with the principles and practices of Mohandas Gandhi, the man who changed a planet with his commitment to nonviolence. Gandhi himself states that his path "calls for strength and courage to suffer without retaliation, to receive blows without returning any" (quoted in Merton, 1996, p. 137). He goes further, however, and notes that this does not exhaust the expectations: "Silence becomes cowardice when occasion demands speaking out the whole truth and acting accordingly" (Merton, 1996, p. 137). What he essentially posits is that nonviolence, interpersonal or otherwise, only becomes a practice when I create the conditions for violence toward myself and, if it comes, elect to not retaliate. This is a hard lesson.

Revisiting manipulation, what I began to understand is that there are two interrelated impulses that make manipulation an attractive option. The first is that it simply makes it possible for one to avoid revealing unpleasant but true things. The second is that should one tell the truth, one could evoke interpersonal violence. That alone can be deeply disturbing. In addition, the desire to retaliate may feel overwhelming. Better to just avoid the whole thing with a gracious manipulation.

And that of course is what many people have asked me: Isn't it better to "keep the peace" through manipulation than precipitate the potential for violence? There is even a lurking sense that doing this "peacekeeping" may be quite virtuous. As is perhaps apparent, Gandhi would not concur if the issue were one of import. The deceit of manipulation is no less deceitful because I hope to avoid interpersonal violence . . . or even more compelling, to avoid the call to the courage of nonretaliation. I have noticed that this doesn't make people want to rush out and discard their manipulative behaviors, and I don't blame them.

I have to admit I am with all the nervous people on this. I often don't know if I have the courage to accept interpersonal violence without retaliation. Gandhi would say that this is a spiritual practice. Perhaps that is the most powerful insight of all. As he would observe, "morality is contraband in war" (Merton, 1996, p. 128). The call to moral courage is not an easy one.

My second caveat focuses on "the South." Raised in the Midwest, I think I had some fairly naïve assumptions about our southern tier of states. I actually thought the Civil War was ancient history. Here, among the southerners, I learned it can also be called the War of Northern Aggression, and that the wounds inflicted by the war are not yet healed. This persistent state of affairs provides an excellent example of the impact of the nonresolution or ineffective resolution of conflict. Because the victor claims that the war is over does not assure that the war is over, as the interlude between World War I and World War II clearly demonstrated.

At a national level, this nonresolution can be described as a cluster of states within a larger federation that remains in many ways "apart," tenaciously maintaining a set of convictions and beliefs about the northern aggressors and the preferred "way of life" of the South. I owe several southerners a debt of gratitude for teaching me how this looks at the personal level. While the observations that follow are generalizations with acknowledged exceptions, the examples themselves are useful.

The southern "way of life," among other things, places a high priority on honor, even honor at a great cost. One thus honors the ways of the South. One also elects to differ with the ways of the North, largely as a matter of principle and with a deep conviction that the ways of the South are "better." This pattern was set during the post–Civil War era, the time of the carpetbaggers when the South experienced itself as a "country" occupied by hostile forces. To have consented to the influences of the North would be tantamount to participating in one's own demeanment.

Here in the South the women's movement sometimes seems to not yet have "happened," and many subtle expressions of racism persist. Southern graciousness is an art form, and its authenticity, while perhaps not personal in nature, is a culturally congruent expectation. These are expressions of those "old ways," and keeping to the old ways is honorable. To do otherwise is to dishonor oneself, to become one with the "enemy."

Hence, manipulation abounds: How to keep the Yankees at bay while maintaining southern honor. To suggest a departure from manipulation is a bit like telling Charlton Heston to turn in his arsenal. It is not merely a personal choice, but a question of fidelity to a culture within a culture. Among woman, this is instructive. The forceful and outspoken women of the East Coast who spear-headed the women's movement will find little congruence between their message and the actions of many, perhaps most southern women. While there are many strong southern women, their style is substantially different from the direct and sometimes abrasive expressions of strength in the North. It is also noteworthy that there is variance in how white women and black women express their strength in the South.

Of course, as I noted, these are generalizations; there are excep-tions. Yet the desire to maintain a culture persists. The unhealed wounds evoke suspicious responses to the Yankee advising a change. This goes beyond the simple struggle of a personal growth option. It seems noteworthy.

Both of these caveats snuggle in the context of a country where political life involves giving everything a "spin" and the role of the media is to try and translate that "spin" and see if it worked. Public discourse, perhaps best exemplified most recently in the presidential election of 2000, leaves one with the sense that the uses of manipulation are multiple and complex. They are internalized and then acted upon as if most citizens were readily manipulated. It is the interaction behavior of choice. This attach-ment to manipulation may be far more ingrained than meets the eye. Why tell the truth when manipulation is such a handy device? Indeed, people who refuse to manipulate others can be judged fools or even unkind.

I continue the search for the fire, continue to seek discernment, and yet find myself sobered by the depth of our attachment to manipulation. I wrote about manipulation as deception and injus-tice, thinking such motives would appear inherently unattractive. What I have since learned is that our dependence on this pattern of behavior is deep and habitual, and that makes the challenge of truth telling even greater. Nonetheless, I persist. It is my hope, I suppose, that others will persist with me.

10

Masks of Manipulation

Manipulation has many faces. It is a wardrobe of masks, and it is indeed artful. To manipulate well is a skill. Many people work years to refine it. To know how to use these masks well provides artful access to control not readily acquired through direct dominance. It can achieve unjust ends with as much success, and sometimes with more. While I do not consider my descriptions of the masks of manipulation exhaustive, they may serve to clarify the meaning of these masks. I have listed ten.

1. Praise and Flattery

Persons accustomed to exercising dominant power without challenges to the legitimacy of this exercise become accustomed to viewing themselves as excelling in the arena where they exercise this power. If they do so in ways that others experience as inappropriate, and they do not permit a challenge to this dominant power, then those being controlled search for ways to equalize the situation, to "get even." One of the easiest approaches is to feed the need of such a person for continuous approval.

People who exercise dominant power inappropriately or to excess do so out of a myriad of motives. It is, however, a fairly safe bet that they are often simply too insecure to do otherwise, that they need to control others to sustain a fragile sense of adequacy. Hence, by praising and flattering them, I can achieve substantial control over the dominators. A truly successful use of this model can even create dependencies on this praise and flattery. Many marriages manifest this. A casual survey of women's magazines will substantiate the fact that it is often the recommended model of choice: "get a man dependent on your praise and flattery, and you can get anything you want from him."

There is of course an implicit insult in this approach, but if a person values vanity, it is easy to "use" praise and flattery. In our culture, we even try to defend it as courtesy or civility, or try to prove it must be used by demonstrating the negative effects of rudeness. We posit that the only way to avoid rudeness is to praise and flatter. We lack the imagination to find ways to be both honest and kind.

We also tend to confuse praise and flattery used manipulatively with genuine nurturance and compassion. This prohibits us from manifesting these profound human qualities when they might be of value to everyone. Praise and flattery can also be used to give the appearance of these qualities, by feigning unqualified acceptance of behaviors in others that would best be confronted and challenged as harmful or destructive. This makes people who use praise and flattery manipulatively seem virtuous and kind, when indeed they may simply be lazy and irresponsible.

2. Lying and Deception

Where praise and flattery fail, lying and deception often enter the dialogue. If I can't flatter you into giving me what I want, I may simply escalate the manipulative cycle and actually lie to you. Sisela Bok (1978) has written, for me, the definitive book on lying. I encourage you to slog through her analysis if this is your favorite model of manipulation.

We like to think lying always involves an active distortion of the truth. It need not be. It can also be done by withholding needed information, or presenting information in such a way that a predicted outcome can be achieved. If the person exercising dominant power reveals a specific vulnerability, I can present facts that impinge on that sense of vulnerability. I can choose to introduce only those facts that will keep the dominant person anxious or uncertain. I can evoke unbalance and then innocently announce that I was merely trying to tell the truth.

I can also pretend I agree with someone exercising dominant power, and then leave the room and announce my disagreement to anyone willing to listen to my story. This is very popular among employees, I think, and was one of the strangest dimensions of being a dean. Even when I would elicit critique and feedback, I would find that people who gave the appearance of concurrence later harshly criticized a decision. When I questioned such people, they assured me that it was because it was impossible to get me to hear their viewpoint. It was often my sense that they simply didn't like my viewpoint and refused to risk "losing" by presenting their own in public.

A variant of this pattern is to defend deception by accusing others of intimidation. In this pattern, I acknowledge that I deceive powerful others, noting that I would have told the truth but the powerful others were intimidating me. I may even contend that this is a justification for my interpersonal violence toward these powerful others. It is perhaps a truism that to differ with persons whom I perceive as more powerful than me can be frightening. To posit that this fear is someone's else's fault, and that it proves the other intended to intimidate me may simply be a complex expression of shadow projection. It can appear to excuse my inaction. It also, however, removes my options of self agency and honest self-reflection. It is costly in that in the effort to deceive others, I concurrently may have deceived myself.

Exaggeration and overstating one's case are also useful variants on lying and deception. These are popularized in legal procedures in this country, especially when winning prevails over an interest in justice. It is not difficult to manipulate the rules of conduct in a courtroom so that clarifications of an exaggeration are silenced as "not germane," creating a deliberate distortion of the truth. While these are sophisticated and subtle manifestations of lying, they are no less lies for their intricacy.

3. Helpfulness and Generosity

I have to admit that this is truly one of my favorites, and I have overused it to the point of nausea on occasion. It has the added value of looking virtuous, in contrast to lying and deception, and thus has a certain appeal for me. It is, however, manipulative if the motive is deception, injustice, or artifice. Like praise and flattery, the intent of the person involved in the behavior is the touchstone.

I'm not real thrilled that I have to reveal that I like this one so much; I think this list could get pretty hard to face without an occasional nod at such human frailty. These types of manipulation are easier to face if you can start acknowledging that you even like some of them. It is also clarifying to note that some may look pretty good on the outside. The real measure of manipulation is the intent of the manipulator. That intent, however, may or may not be conscious. That is why it is so disconcerting when someone kills you with kindness. It offends you rather than pleasing you. It can even, over time, make you homicidal. I should know; I'm pretty sure I've been on several hit lists.

One of the artifices of helpfulness and generosity is that it often has an "IOU" attached; giving is done in the hope that guilt alone will lead to returns, that one can shame a person exercising dominant power into giving in return, or giving in. Many religious systems in our country support this artifice, while failing to explore the deceit implicit in the process. We have been bargaining with one or another god for many centuries.

The deceit nestles in the intent, the danger in the outcome. If this "works," what it tells those exercising dominant power is that the price that they can extract for giving is the requirement of helpfulness and generosity. Thus, the artifice of the manipulator becomes the currency of the exchange, and the person exercising dominant power simply escalates the expectations. The national dependency on wealthy women as unpaid volunteers for civic development is a wonderful example of this dynamic institutionalized and normalized. Its seduction is of course the wonderful sense of virtuousness that it creates for everyone.

This particular manipulative maneuver also reveals one of the reasons why it is so difficult to discriminate about manipulation. I may not have developed enough self-awareness yet to know that I am being manipulative, that my helpfulness has a hook attached. Then, when I discover it, I may find I don't want to behave manipulatively anymore, and hence refuse to be helpful and generous. I may think that the behavior itself is the issue, rather than my motives. Hence, not only is the habituation to manipulation a challenge, but even after I have greater clarity in my understanding of manipulative behaviors, transforming the behavior may introduce further challenges. No wonder we all stay so stuck.

4. Trickery and Secret Deals

Another equally normalized variant on manipulation is the creating of secret deals that contaminate the public negotiation with behind-the-scenes agreements that determine the outcome. The public negotiation is simply a charade. This is most popularized in our current model of political discourse, where the assumption of integrity or honesty is viewed as suspect, outside the norm. Indeed, the popular media largely now focus on the fairly cynical search for the "real deal" behind the charade, and call this the news. We assume the secret deal has been cut, and call it inevitable, as if we were incapable of doing otherwise. We effectively reinforce our collective capacity to be at our worst.

Such deals are often supported with the assertion that they are necessary, that there is no other choice, that human nature being what it is, we have to pander to the lowest common denominator. It is a great deal easier for us to be at our worst than to be at our best. That we structure to sustain this ease is less compelling.

If indeed we accept secret deals and trickery as normal, we can then discover an endless array of alternatives for negotiating toward base instincts. This does not require a visionary. We can even, if we feel the dominant power is quite awful, manipulate a negotiation so that the process fails, or prevails with frank dishonesty. I find this particular form of manipulation unattractive but have found myself repeatedly attracted to the idea of using it—then manifesting something other than the deal cut when it goes public. Since the whole thing is tainted, acting otherwise seems stupid, and revealing the dishonesty seems attractive. Having tried this a few times in a modest way, it is my experience that this can really upset a person with dominant power. If upsetting is the goal, it really works. See how easy it is to get into pursuing base instincts.

The obvious danger is one of limits: once secret deals and trickery become the norm, the limits are unclear. Thus, this manipulation can be used not only to craft dishonest and polluted political deals, but to reveal them and use this revelation to discredit the dominant power. Both uses, however, tend to exacerbate rather than solve conflicts in a situation of unequal power. Obviously, if our basest instincts become normative, we can pursue a course of ever-expanding depravity in the name of human nature. Unbridled violence in our culture is an instructive exemplar. If we use trickery and secret deals to create the laws of the land, and to defend them in courts of purported justice, it is little wonder that we do not sense the moral persuasion of the law.

5. Attacking and Threatening

This form of manipulation has the charm of instant familiarity. It is popular at nearly every uneven table. It takes on the dominant power and tries to equalize the situation by simply exercising counterdominant power. Saul Alinsky's *Rules for Radicals* (1971) often used this model, albeit with very clever versions of this behavior. His book was one of the first to shape my thinking about inequality, and it has taken me some time to find the darknesses in his model since much of it seems wise. Attacking and threatening simply continue the fixation on dominant power. They also tend to escalate the conflict. They implicitly tell persons who are inappropriately exercising dominant power that they should and must continue to do so to protect themselves from the manipulator. This one just doesn't work in the long run.

There are more subtle versions of this, however. These are often very personal in nature, and attack and threaten not about the issue at hand, but about the personal worth of the person exercising dominant power. They point out frailties in others and use this to diminish their credibility. I think one of the best books available on how women further this dynamic is Jean Baker Miller's *Toward a New Psychology of Women* (1976). Gordon Allport also captures some of this dynamic in *The Nature of Prejudice* (1958). Both authors unveil some of the secondary effects of sustaining inequality over time and the disturbed relationships that emerge. If attacking and threatening are personal in nature, one can upset the persons with dominant power, activate insecurity, and get them to function ineffectively. This can involve baiting, coercing, and badgering.

The fact that this particular face of manipulation is so commonplace warrants further reflection. At first blush, it appears to merely be the use of dominant power to confront dominant power. To qualify as a manipulative maneuver, however, it must embrace some degree of artifice, deceit, or injustice. Often the artifice used is to proclaim that the attack or the threat was valid because a counterpressure to the exercise of dominant power was needed. All of this appears to argue that the only currency available is dominant power. It actually demonstrates that fear, intimidation, activation of guilt, shaming, humiliating, belittling, discounting, slander, and libel are also useful currencies. Thus, this manipulation can wear the face of virtue or honest combat and actually be quite another thing. If motives are denied or distorted, the face of manipulation rears its ugly head.

Time-Out

This list is pretty hard to take in. Because dominant power in our culture is so oversubscribed, just about everyone has developed a fairly well-honed set of manipulative skills designed to help them get by and get even. These manipulative skills may be unreflective behaviors, and they may create a life without much joy, bliss, or ecstasy, but they are familiar and we have become accustomed to them. We kind of hate to see them just up and leave the room.

Laziness keeps us from growing out of these, but there are other reasons, too. We may not want to study these faces of manipulation because if we look too long and hard at our own dark sides, we may begin to feel like that's all that's there. Shadows scare us. We may be willing to see the various forms of manipulation in others more readily than in ourselves, but again fear that that's all that's there. We lose touch with the magnificent and profound dimensions of humanity when we overemphasize the darknesses. Keeping a balance is a challenge.

That's why I called a time-out. You've actually slogged your way through only half of this list. But we could all use some balance time. The only way I'm able to honestly look at my dark side is to make sure I give equal attention to the dimensions of me that I experience as more mature, wise, courageous, beautiful, temperate, loving, compassionate, and honest. When I have trouble locating these dimensions in myself, I try to remember that I'm part of a larger creation, and turn to that creation to remind me of these dimensions of life on this planet, of which I am a part.

I'm living in Galveston, Texas, as I write this book. My home is three blocks from a peaceful stretch of Gulf of Mexico beach, and it is my place of balancing. Galveston is a barrier reef island with magnificent sunrises and sunsets, moon rises and moon sets. These are reminders. The tempo in Galveston is slow and temperate, matching daily temperatures and breezes from the Gulf. These are the rhythms I try to learn from, watching the tidal pull shaping waves, washing ashore both the detritus and the life forms of the Gulf. Spidery boats dot the Gulf horizon when some special fish are running, and then for days the boats virtually disappear from view. We celebrate Mardi Gras in a frenzy and seem virtually quiescent during gray winds of January. I live in a resort development. On weekends, my neighborhood is abuzz with folks from Houston who "come down" to visit the island; on weekdays, my life seems hermetic, and I am surrounded by silent homes devoid of human life.

These are the rhythms of planetary life, human and otherwise, that remind me that there are both a dark and a light side to being human, that most of my existence is about rhythms and cycles, and that I can sustain a long hard look at the darkness if I can keep in mind that the light will dawn. I also have learned, over time, that I do not benefit from clinging to the light. It is in the darkness that I learn lessons that the light cannot teach. The moon on the Gulf is no less beautiful than the sun; it is merely different. Life would be poorer for me without these dark lesson times. It is in this spirit that I think one might best study a list of hard things to face.

An Exercise

Now that I've shared with you some of the ways I search for, cling to, discover, or rediscover balance when I'm struggling for self-honesty and courage, I thought a brief exercise might be in order. This one goes in your journal. Just writing the heading "Time-Out from Manipulation" will help you imagine that you could actually take such a time-out.

This exercise gives you a chance to distract yourself from all these negative pictures and shift your gaze to some balancing positive pictures. You may have recognized yourself in one of those negative pictures, and if you didn't you may be pretty worried about your level of denial. Here are some images to conjure up before you continue to look at the rest of the picture.

Write down what you think are your five best traits. Head the list thus: "My Five Best Traits." Imprint these for a moment. Remember that you have them. If one of them might really be manipulative, try an alternate. See, in addition to drifting off into mindless manipulation, you also have some good qualities that might be useful at an uneven table.

Conjure up and then write down the names of five people you admire. Title the list "Five Really Great People." Beside each name, write down the quality that you most admire in this person. Imprint these for a minute. If one of the qualities is actually manipulative, try an alternate. Isn't it nice to know that there are some wonderful things out there to discover in humans besides their capacity for manipulation? You might even find some of these operative at an uneven table and might want to emulate them.

Conjure up and then write down five beautiful things. Head the list as follows: "Five Beautiful Things." There are no rules here. Imprint them, recall them, try to feel and experience them. If some are immediately available, go and experience them: a partner, a moving rendition of a song, a painting, a bowl of chili. Celebrate them, enjoy them, laugh at the sheer joy of them.

It is useful to recall that whenever I cringe at the challenge of self-honesty or search in vain for the courage to change, I always have at least these fifteen things to call on to keep me in balance if I start to get weird and negative. Keep these lists. Someday, try for ten, or, in a moment of wild abandon, try twenty or two hundred. If you get very good at this, you might be amazed at how much self-honesty and courage you can try for when the positive lists are so nice and long.

As you might have guessed, it's time to go back to the faces of manipulation.

6. Deliberate Stupidity

I didn't really plan it this way, but if you didn't do that last exercise, you may have just turned yourself into an audiovisual aid for this face of manipulation. This mask is one of the trickier ones to grasp, since those who use it regularly have the greatest difficulty understanding it. I assume this doesn't really surprise you. Actually, if you like this version of manipulation, you may succeed in failing to understand this entire section of the book.

If you're very deeply attached to using manipulation as a problem-solving device, anything that challenges you to face your manipulative behavior can become pretty threatening. When all else fails, you can just not get it, become confused, or wander aimlessly in soliloquies about obtuse points of difference, fail to understand. There is something wonderfully effective about this form of manipulation. Students love it.

And persons exercising dominant power do not love it. I have found it to be very effective with me when I am inappropriately exercising dominant power. I get easily waylaid into trying to explain my reason for exercising power to the point of idiocy, while the manipulator gives me a pleasant but confused, often blank facial expression. The most effective manifestation of this is for the manipulator to then say, "I just don't get it." My daughters, during their teen years, taught me that deliberate stupidity can even be effective when I am appropriately exercising dominant power. I have great respect for this mode of manipulation.

What this may reveal is that the form you least like to use yourself may indeed be the one most effectively used to manipulate you. I like to appear intelligent, even when I'm not all that sure I'm on the right road. Hence, deliberate stupidity does not appeal to me as a mode of manipulation. It therefore is very effective with me, because it feels very controlling and I haven't a clue about how to end the impasse. Using this type of manipulation effectively makes it impossible to bring the conflict to a resolution. As is apparent, I hope, the hook in this dynamic is not merely someone else's deliberate stupidity, but my vanity.

There are secondary gains in this approach that are worth mentioning. If I am too stupid to understand the issues, I in effect absent myself from any responsibility for solving the problem. We who lack the ability simply cannot help out. Of course, one also then absents oneself from the opportunity to engage in creative problem solving, to grow and mature, to generate more effective ways of living. But the gains are there to be had, dishonest and limiting as they prove to be.

7. Cuteness and Flirtatiousness

I was two heads taller than most of my classmates in eighth grade, so I never fully mastered this skill. It's hard to look down at short guys and try to be cute at the same time. They seemed to like me and considered me a good friend but rarely viewed me as cute, thus effectively discouraging any drift I felt toward flirtatiousness. Yet I have seen this

form of manipulation used so effectively that I feel it merits a category of its own. It is a favorite of many women but, contrary to popular wisdom, is also used by men. I have modified it modestly to suit
my ends with the use of cleverness and wittiness. These work as well
at least at distracting, and sometimes at signaling that all that dominant power can turn into mush with minimal effort.

Flirtatiousness and seduction are modes of manipulation that do
their harm in a more personal way and tend to touch pockets of
human vulnerability in others that are often less easily mastered or
managed. They rarely focus on the issues of a conflict, rarely alter
the distribution of dominant power at an uneven table; but they do
upset the focus of the power. If someone is trying to exercise inappropriate control over me, changing the subject can almost always
distract for the moment. To seduce or flirt deceitfully may distract
with a vengeance. The ensuing dynamics that emerge, depending
on the depth and scope of the seduction, can wreak serious havoc
with the lives of those visited with this form of manipulation. They
can also return to harm the seducer with a vengeance.

This is a poorly explored area in our culture, in part because we
are collectively experiencing cataclysmic changes in gender relationships that none of us fully understand. We are also struggling
with a myriad of conflicting thoughts and feelings about sexuality
and friendship, and a deep uncertainty about how to create effective relationships across and within fragmented gender boundaries.
In our confusion, we are perhaps even more susceptible to the lure
of seduction, the hope that something pleasing is occurring, the
desire that something positive will emerge.

Often seduction and flirting are accompanied by flattery, which
activates our need for admiration or heightened self-esteem. Under
these conditions, this manipulative tool, so powerful in its long-
term effects in the personal lives of individuals, can seem to have a
unique utility and charm. Perhaps for that reason, it is all the more
damaging in the long run, both to those who use it and to those
who are the object of the manipulation. These behaviors are also

actively reinforced and valued in our culture, making it difficult to recognize when they may prove harmful and dangerous.

8. Perseverating

This one is my all-time favorite, and no matter how I write about it, it will be clear that I cling to it like a teddy bear in the night. I think it is the primary tool used by every nurse fighting for what she or he believes to be the best or right thing to do, and believing that no other tool is available. It is a mask, but a powerful one compared to some of the other options on this list. It doesn't resolve conflicts— it often worsens them—but it can get you things you can't seem to get any other way, so it is seductive in its appeal.

I hope you just noticed how easy it is for me to defend this obvious form of manipulation. This is one of the problems with manipulations. They seem like the best or only solution. They get you something in the short run. They work once and you want to keep on using them. They have an allure about them. It is harder to note and admit that they do harm, sustain conflicts, do not alter the nature of the discourse about dominant power, and can in the long run create a situation that permits others to continue to discount or belittle you.

If you perseverate, you hang on to an issue long enough to outlast the best of the crowd. You "keep bringing it up." You repeat the theme song until people get so worn down by it that they'll do anything for the privilege of switching channels. It has subsets: harping and nagging. I suddenly imagine my children saying "Yup, that's Mom!" This is not comforting. I also realize that since I have shown such slow progress in giving up harping, nagging, and perseverating, wanting to continue to defend them, cling to them, and find a false security in them, I am particularly vulnerable to people using them with me. I overreact, overrespond, and give in, no doubt out of guilt. I hope my children are still reading. It would comfort me to know that they read this part too.

Perseveration does not alter the situation; it merely overreacts to one dimension of a situation. It does not generate creative alternatives to an unequal table; it accommodates unequal tables and inadvertently strengthens the existing structures. It gives the appearance of succeeding but fails to create a new paradigm. Because I am clinging to it still, however, I would like to tell you perseverators out there that I know just how you feel. Unfortunately, we're wrong.

9. Withholding

There are a variety of ways of expressing the manipulative face of withholding: passive aggression, pouting, forced silence, withdrawal. Each freezes the process of negotiation by disengagement. No outcome can be achieved because no progress can be made. It essentially exercises countercontrol by withdrawal, inaction, absence, the refusal to participate. Because it does not involve an overt action, it has the added attraction of presenting itself as innocent and pure. Sometimes it is even viewed or presented as principled or reflective, as in "still waters run deep." Some still water is just stagnant—an alternate view that cannot be tested if the silence is sustained and the passivity is a well-honed skill.

The balance between activity and passivity is one of life's great mysteries and challenges. I personally find it eludes me much of the time, more than most challenges. It is a difficult rhythm to discover and sustain. Both have their intrinsic place in life. Thus, when passivity does emerge, especially in a culture active to the point of frenzy, it can have a certain calming effect, an appeal, even evoke a respect. Sometimes that respect is also appropriate. When passivity is used to deceive, its virtue is tainted. Like other forms of manipulation, intent clarifies. If the motive is deceptive in nature, passivity becomes manipulation.

The appeal of passivity, for me, is that I don't have to do much. I can just sit here like a lichen on a log. I can even practice saying some pleasant sentences as needed, to appear engaged. Others may perceive me as "going along" even though I have made no commitments, embrace no obligations. Then, I absolve myself from any responsibility. After all, I just "was there"; I didn't actually say I agreed. My male colleagues in academe have often shared with me their frustration at the number of times their female colleagues have used this form of manipulation. This may simply indicate that I use it infrequently. Perhaps they are telling my more passive female colleagues about how irritating my perseverating can be.

I tend to think of this as the low-energy-expenditure manipulation, the least imaginative of the lot. In a culture compelled toward more and more complexity and propelled toward higher and higher speeds of activity, it can, however, have a substantial impact. Withholding can successfully disrupt even the most effective effort at the exercise of dominant power. It can seem soothing and comforting and therefore seductive. It can then, effectively, "get its way" and thus enjoys more popularity than the silence and withdrawal might at first predict.

10. Obeisance

I think I used the word obeisance here because it sounds like it feels to me: sort of oily and clinging and fake. It might equally have been called compliance or obedience or submission or cooptation. All imply a dimension of the process of giving up and giving in, of going along, of being coopted. They do not adequately capture the dimension of doing so "for inside control," however. The obeisant manipulator goes along deceitfully, with an intent to get something from the "deal."

It is difficult to discuss this manipulation, since it introduces a whole new range of options for people who have simply been going along and giving up, obedient and submissive as if there were no other options. The obeisant person, however, recognizes that if submission is required, it will have a price tag. There are many ways of extracting one's pound of flesh. This type of manipulation is perhaps a variant on secret deals, but it is even sneakier, since the obeisant person never fully reveals that a price will be extracted later on. It simply emerges over time.

Obeisance has the advantage of engaging the dominant power over time, of permitting one to stay at the table forever, of always being certain of getting something back, albeit through deceit. It is one of the more confounding manipulations, since it reinforces the belief that the best way to make gains is to be co-opted. The rewards will be secret, but they will at least be there. This approach also highlights the lack of obeisance of all the others at an uneven table, who are then often cast in a darker and more troublesome light. It is not one of my favorite manipulations, both because it seems to extract such a high personal price and because of the burden it places on others.

The Key to a Sound Manipulation

It may be helpful at this point to see the ten masks of manipulation as a composite, sort of like a menu for deceit and injustice. For each, the intention to deceive and perpetrate injustice is the basis for action. Since motive is central, we are unable to judge their presence in the behaviors of others with certainty. We do, however, have the option of evaluating our own intentions if we elect to do so. Here's the list:

Praise and flattery

Lying and deception

Helpfulness and generosity

Trickery and secret deals

Attacking and threatening

Deliberate stupidity

Cuteness and flirtatiousness

Perseverating

Withholding

Obeisance

Not a pretty picture. The key to sustaining all of these manipulations at an uneven table is self-deception. That is why it is so difficult to read about them. Reading about them can disrupt a nice tidy pattern of self-deception. It has actually been pretty hard to write about them. I'm always startled at how frequently I turn a corner and find one more form of self-deception just lurking there, waiting for me with a silly grin on its face.

Since all manipulations involve deceit and injustice, if one goes to an uneven table and wishes to claim others are deceitful or unjust, it is somewhat ineffective to do so by acting out various forms of deceit and injustice. This is nice and tidy and logical but does not dramatically alter human behavior. Despite the lack of logic in our actions, we persist.

Hence, these popularized forms of deceit are often sustained by trying to convince ourselves that we don't engage in such heinous behaviors. The sell job is a difficult one, and we often fail at it, but we persist in trying. The projection of our shadow side may be difficult, but it is striking how willing we are to work hard at the challenge. As is perhaps obvious to you by now, this naming of the problem is a pretty messy business, and makes sorting the dirty laundry, in comparison, quite appealing. At least we know how to turn it into clean folded laundry. If we are indeed invested in keeping our linen dirty, it is hard to get access to the feelings of satisfaction that come from folding all those fluffy, clean towels, shirts, and underwear.

Mold

Banquet scraps grow green in cold storage,
bringing catalytic recall in domestic forages.
Foamy swipes half greet the surging memories
stacked on counters in faces bland as Tupperware.

Decisions are made at the garbage disposal;
furry assaults on the universe, diluted and ground.
Lake Michigan will absorb me yet, one way or another;
the dishwasher is full of recycled containers.

There is a stream to all this uncollected garbage.
There are crude ceremonies for all this letting out.
My daughters are still generating leftovers.
I eat everything on my plate.
—pbk

Manipulation: Summary

I imagine that you are pleased to have survived reading the list of manipulation exemplars. They are uncomfortable, but not merely because we feel a tug of denial, hoping to sustain our self-deceptions. Inherently, if we listen to our own best instincts, we know that these behaviors have some things in common.

They all successfully sustain the role of victim and enable others to sustain the role of victimizer. They actually perpetuate a cycle, where each participant eventually will play both roles. All victimizers eventually become victims, and all victims eventually become victimizers. All these behaviors also involve substantial secondary gains. People get attached to them and learn to rely on them. They are lifestyles. In some cases, they can be virtually addictive.

They are also "rewarded" behaviors in some fashion or another. They help others play and sustain a role of "superior" person. They assume that the inappropriate exercise of dominant power is so unchangeable that one best addresses this by adapting through manipulation, and getting whatever gains can be had from the situation. Since the person exercising dominant power inappropriately is to some degree captured in an illusion, this illusion is thereby strengthened and sustained.

The various masks of manipulation also require, at least to some degree, the temporary suppression of feelings. In addition to the obvious impact that suppressed feelings have on general well-being, the masks add the threat of these feelings eventually reemerging to further exacerbate what is now an already troublesome dynamic. They are all harmful in nature.

I personally was taught all of these modes of manipulation, sometimes several times over. I've been rewarded for most of them at some point in my lifetime. I've also been the object of all of them. I have even sometimes rewarded people for using them on me. Yet no one really seems to think they're all that great. We don't really want this to be the best we can do. Still, we seem to believe we lack options.

Most of these types of manipulation are now so common that we have normalized them, called them human nature, and excused them in ourselves and others like one might excuse the inability to walk on water or speak twelve languages fluently: "We humans simply can't do better," we mutter. We believe them to be a given of human nature rather than a clumsy and destructive substitute for more constructive, creative, and personally satisfying behaviors.

Often discussions about conflict resolution assume the presence of such behaviors. Some of these behaviors are even offered as tools to the negotiator. The goal in such cases is not necessarily injustice, but it may be deceit. Intentionality is not always that easy to ascertain, self-deception is often compelling, and the outcome is a set of behaviors in a negotiator that clearly furthers the conflict.

More often, however, conflict resolution proponents identify these behaviors as "problem behaviors" that need to be dealt with, mitigated, even manipulated. Often the labeling of the behaviors as "problematic" is a short circuit in determining the basis for the behavior. If a person becomes manipulative, it might at least be interesting to find out if that person is experiencing the table of negotiation as uneven.

A Story

For several years, I have taught psychiatric nursing. It is a wonderful specialty in nursing, where I have always felt I've had endless opportunities to improve the lives of others and at least in one small space and time, to make a difference. I enjoy teaching it and have enjoyed even more students who make discoveries that mirror my own.

One such student once cared for an adolescent female who had been hospitalized for depression and suicidal behavior. She was being closely watched for these self-harming tendencies, but the real focus of interest for most of her caregivers was the fact that for three weeks she had refused to take a shower or bath. This had become something of a unit-wide concern, and the power struggle that ensued was complex. I concluded she had more taste for life than most humans, having mounted a successful three-week campaign to ward off all showermongers in the unit.

The student assigned to her care was a quiet, reflective young woman who felt a natural empathy for this girl and established an easy and gentle relationship with her. After two days of watching the shower "war," the student and I met to discuss the issue. We decided that since the student had a comfortable relationship with the girl, perhaps she could slowly elicit the reason for this refusal.

The student patiently communicated her way to the question. The girl had noticed that people walked in on others who were taking a shower. The place where she was advised to shower lacked natural privacy, and the other showers that might have been available could easily be entered by others. She did not want her privacy violated. It was a simple, honest, and understandable desire. She believed that since people were watching her so closely and knew of her suicidal wishes, they would surely burst in on her in the shower and shame and embarrass her. She knew they had an excuse: she was suicidal.

We set a plan of action. We procured commitments from all persons in decision-making roles to honor our plan. The student would help her get her things into the shower, close the door, and stand guard. She would talk to her through the door occasionally to make sure everything was OK, but she would not enter the shower space. The girl, on the other hand, committed herself to using the time to shower, not to attend to her suicidal thoughts. It was a moment of high drama, and the shower was taken as planned.

The young patient, after her shower, obviously felt better and was reassured that someone would honor her trust. The caregivers in the unit gave her a large dose of congratulations, which she obviously enjoyed. She became more responsive to others and began to make steady progress. The student and I, later, marveled at how little it took to discover so much good under one foolish standoff about dominant power and control.

That this girl had to fight so hard for twenty minutes of privacy, and that no one had found a way to find out what she wanted, seems ridiculous in retrospect—but many power struggles look that way in retrospect. Often we assume that people who behave manipulatively do so because it is their tool of choice, the one that they are convinced will best serve their self-interest. Covertly, unintentionally, this attitude can sustain their behavior and even trap them in it.

An interesting alternative question might be, Why do people use these behaviors? Sometimes it is because they believe that they are negotiating at a table that they know is uneven. Sometimes they know that this fact is ignored, denied, or discounted as insignificant. Sometimes they believe there is nothing that they can do about this, that they lack alternatives. If these conditions exist, they may believe that the only alternative available is manipulation. In our culture, where manipulative behavior is normalized, they may even view this alternative as preferred, desirable, or admirable.

11

Traditional Methods of Maneuvering

The manipulative behaviors I have just described serve as building blocks of a sort, the stones or bricks we use to erect more elaborate structures. Such structures can eventually take on the solidity of a well-designed building and become as common as the houses in our neighborhoods or the stores on our main streets. When these composites of manipulation become solidified, they can become such a predictable part of our lives that we view them not as stylized manipulations, but as "normal" communications or "normal" behaviors. We bring them to an uneven table, and we accept them as the behaviors that people typically manifest in a negotiation. We don't search for alternatives; we expect them and create negotiations that expect them. These composites of manipulation warrant further discussion.

Methods of Maneuvering

Finding yourself at an uneven table stretches manipulation skills. The following descriptions of methods of maneuvering are not exhaustive but help sketch a picture of the scenes one might find when visiting such a table.

I Won't and I Don't Because I Can't

People at an uneven table often literally can't see a place to stand, so they freeze their behavior. If one is accustomed to using manipulative behaviors, these behaviors become even more appealing as one becomes enmeshed in challenging or threatening negotiations about a conflict. Rarely do we adequately pursue such dilemmas long enough or in an open-enough fashion to discover that often people believe that they "can't" do anything but freeze.

Sometimes people at an uneven table will try to articulate their concerns. If they are silenced or their issues are dismissed as untenable or irrelevant, they directly experience a message that says, "You can't." It is then not so surprising that they believe this to be the case. At an uneven table, if someone signals that my concerns are not acceptable or my viewpoint can be disregarded, I can easily find myself believing that I can't achieve my goals or negotiate in an open and constructive fashion.

A Parable

Once upon a time, there was a wonderful country full of wonderful people who believed in freedom. They found many delightful ways to experience and enjoy this freedom, and over time they valued it more and more. They lived, however, near other countries where freedom was not so highly prized, and they felt the need to develop and maintain a plan to protect their freedoms.

They made a careful appraisal of the neighboring countries and noticed that in these other places, killing, war, and destruction were used to keep freedom from happening. They decided they had better be ready for something like that to happen, so they created a plan. If the other countries came to kill, make war, and destroy, they would defend themselves. They too would kill, make war, and destroy as needed.

They of course determined that they needed to select some people who would be in charge of killing, making war, and destroying. They would also need several people to help with the task. As they set out to implement the plan, they discovered that just about everyone was pretty anxious about killing, making war, and destroying other people. They expressed this with a whole collection of other feelings like fear, vulnerability, shame, guilt, revulsion, and panic. Yet the need persisted to solve the potential threat to their freedoms.

They set out to teach all the people who were working on developing the skills for killing, making war, and destroying how to manage these feelings that kept them from their task. They helped all of them stop experiencing these feelings. They helped them deny these feelings. They helped them suppress these feelings. They helped them project these feelings. To be really effective, they discovered it worked best to start the training early, preferably at birth. After a while, they were very successful.

One day, while they were sitting around enjoying their freedoms, they casually asked some of the people trained to kill, make war, and destroy how they "felt" about their freedoms that day. The trained people became very confused. They said what they thought about the freedoms. "No, no, we want to know how you feel about the freedoms!" they replied enthusiastically. The trained persons looked very confused. "Feel, what is feel? We don't know what you are talking about. We don't know what feeling is."

Cynicism

This expression of human despair is so popularized and normalized in our culture that the blunting of human sensibility inherent in it is no longer even acknowledged. On the contrary, it is viewed as a mark of sophistication and intelligence. Persons incapable of cynicism are viewed as foolish, naïve, uninformed, and unwilling to grapple with the inherent nastiness of life. Even the modest effort to state the ironic or sardonic dimensions of a situation is quickly crammed into the assumptions of cynicism.

What cynicism achieves is the collapse of the creative possibilities in human behavior. It constricts and destroys instincts, spirit, and soul, and indeed assumes they do not exist, or that if they do, they are evil or hopeless. It negates intuition, and the aesthetic, and discards the ethical as mere intellectual meandering. It closes the door to trust and candor by flaunting a dishonest version of trust and candor. It harms.

Cynicism is actually an intellectualized version of attack, usually based on discounting and belittling. It is a passive-aggressive ploy. It creates the impression of a commitment to truth by belittling others and positing oneself as practical and realistic. It gets even by diminishing others under the guise of intelligence. It is a favorite tool of the news media in this country, demonstrating an inability to differentiate between cynicism and effective criticism. It is often used in science to deny the existence of any reality other than the physical.

A Story

I am writing this book during a period of cataclysmic change in health care delivery in the United States. It is hard not to notice some linkages between what I'm trying to say here and what is swirling around me on a daily basis in the health care arena.

One major shift that attracts the attention of nurses is the shift to a more visible, comprehensive, and respected role in health care delivery for nurses who have advanced preparation, either as nurse practitioners, certified nurse midwives, nurse anesthetists, or certified clinical specialists. These nurses now provide excellent primary care for individuals, families, and communities. The degree to which they have been able to do so has historically been limited by legislative and political control through the efforts of organized physician groups who have viewed such nursing practice as a threat to their power, wealth, and control. Many members of these groups have essentially abandoned the persons who need this care the most—the poor—and yet they oppose nurses giving the care.

One of the reasons for this opposition is significant. Research has indicated that where nurses deliver this care, their outcomes are as good as and in some cases much better than those of physicians. In the case of nurse midwives, for instance, many physicians have been willing to have these nurses care for indigent women, who often have complex pregnancies. When women who were not indigent sought midwives for this superior level of care, however, physician political groups often worked actively to prohibit it. They have also insisted that they be reimbursed for care at a higher rate than nurses, even when the same care is being provided.

All this appears to be shifting some under proposals emerging with health care reform. Some people want to see advanced-practice nurses given the freedom and responsibility to deliver the quality care they're prepared to deliver without physician intrusion or control. This has upset some physicians.

Only days after several health care reform proposals were announced in the early 90s, the political action committee of one state medical association delivered a poster to all its members. I do not know what the members are supposed to do with the poster. It pictures a group of ducks. The words "quack, quack, quack" are written near the ducks. The poster also advises the viewer to not let reform "fowl up" your health delivery system with the intrusion of persons such as nurse practitioners and nurse midwives. It presents these nurses as forces that would seriously affect the quality of care and do harms, as "quacks." Persistence counts. Ten years later, this issue remains unresolved.

Holding Emotional Hostages

We are all pretty vulnerable humans. Persons at an uneven table who exercise dominant power, both appropriately and inappropriately, are as vulnerable as those who do not. We can prey on that vulnerability. We can cut emotional deals that create dependencies. We can appear to be trying to help them with their emotional vulnerability but actually be preying on it.

It is not difficult to persuade persons that we meet their needs. If they experience even moderate levels of normal human emotional vulnerability, having their needs met can feel good. We can then convince them that they need us, that they can't negotiate without us. If they believe this, they will begin to be more vulnerable, and we can convince them that we can't negotiate without them. Then, having successfully created a mutual dependency, we can hold them hostage emotionally. Inevitably, in such a negotiation, we will find that we too are held hostage.

We can also withhold our honest reactions from dominant persons, tell them we agree with them, suppress our differences or our resentments that they are controlling us, and assure them that we think that they are wonderful and good and true. We can inflate their egos so dramatically that they become unable to deal with situations where a more realistic picture of their worth is presented. Such a maneuver can create dependency on the distorted message, and one is then an emotional hostage. Persons being controlling can become so dependent that they make all their choices in the light of sustaining this message. As is obvious, they are then not in control but are being controlled.

Fear

Catalytic timid lies
spark passage to remember;
no forgiveness, no reprise,
relentless white December.

Banal sketches of defeat,
pernicious as debate:
no encampment, no retreat,
a spiraling of hate.

  —pbk

Humoring the Fools

We can achieve a semblance of covert and false parity by becoming supercilious about those exercising dominant power and humor them along, deceiving them the whole way. We can work hard to convince them that we are on their side, while covertly we are "laughing up our sleeve." We say one thing to their face, another when they are absent. This behavior diminishes everyone; it is a variant of cynicism.

Since many times in this book I have used examples that demonstrate the frustration and limitations experienced by nurses who confront physicians who exercise dominant power well beyond what is either rational or desirable, it seems fair at this juncture to honestly state the "other side" of this story. Nurses have accommodated this injustice far too often using this behavior as the dynamic of choice. Nurses have been humoring physicians for decades, and the outcomes have been harmful to everyone. I am not saying this with pride or even false humility, but it deserves an honest statement, since the costs for everyone have been high.

A Story

As a young nurse, I worked for a year in a surgical department, primarily either assisting in specific surgical procedures as a "scrub nurse" (one who actually scrubs for a case) or as a "circulating nurse"—a nurse available to the surgical team to bring in sterile supplies, alter equipment, and keep the progression of the surgery environmentally supported. I was a good scrub nurse and was sought after for the job. I was also flattered by this fact.

One Saturday afternoon a physician needed to apply a cast to a small girl, nine months old. The cast was to extend from midchest to her ankles, covering both legs. These casts were hard to apply, and a wiggling nine-month-old child complicates the challenge. We had a cast room in the surgical suite, and the physician came there to apply the cast, asking me to assist him. My supervisor concurred.

I had a conviction as a nurse that it was important to always communicate with patients as much as possible during preparations for surgical procedures or during them. It was known that I did this, and while I was often teased for doing so, it was clear to me and everyone else that it helped to relax the patients. So I proceeded as usual.

I had placed the little girl on a crib and stood opposite the physician, who was preparing to apply the cast. I enveloped the little girl in my arms and placed my face very close to hers and began to say soft, soothing things to her. She slowly relaxed and was transfixed by the process, unmindful of the casting activity going on. We were in a warm communication, and she was peaceful and still.

The physician was one I respected and enjoyed, a competent and principled man with a good sense of humor. He began teasing me about my communication with this child. I was carefully trying to ignore him and stay focused on the child. As I ignored him, his teasing escalated. He was enjoying himself and was relaxed because the squirmy little nine-month-old girl was as peaceful as a summer lake.

I continued ignoring him and the teasing escalated even more. We neared the end. I suddenly reacted to some comment, broke my concentration on the little girl, and returned one of his salvos with one of my own. I wanted to prove myself clever, perhaps to defend myself and my skill, perhaps merely to show that I too could verbally spar with the best of them. I wanted to respond. As I did so, the little girl startled, wiggled, then howled, then thrashed. The cast went into contortions, the procedure had to be redone, and I learned the shame of abandoning a patient to humor the fools.

Emotional Numbing and Deadening

If we go to an uneven table, we come there as feeling humans, ones who experience emotion. We will quickly discover that some of the things that persons with dominant power say and do hurt those feelings. We will discover that the assumption that we are inferior or are to be treated unjustly as if it were acceptable is itself hurtful. This is human pain of a certain sort that often feels best simply denied, since we are often unable to find some way of mitigating the pain.

We may learn to silence, dismiss, delete, suppress, or never again feel our feelings. Then we don't hurt so much, we believe, and we can stay at the table, participating in the negotiation. What we often fail to realize is that in doing so, we also deaden our capacity to discriminate feelings—both our own and those of others—and to empathize. We begin to distort and to destroy and don't even know that we are doing so.

Impeccable

Did the shadows then protect you?
Did the masks reduce your pain?
Did you keep your skin unsullied?
Did you not melt in the rain?
Did you answer all your memos?
Did you silence every song?
Did you dust the plastic flowers?
Then I'm sure you did no wrong.

—pbk

Some Lies Are Okay Because I Mean Well

Confusion about means and ends is one of those irritating moral realities that never abates. Even with lies, we flounder. We think that we can lie our way to some higher good. The line on lies is hard to draw; once we compromise our sense of the truth, we can never fully retrieve it. We may recover, but not retrieve. The realization that our lie "got us what we wanted" can further impair our ability to recognize the damaging impact of lying, and intensify our commitment to defend our deceptions as acceptable because our intentions were meritorious.

All lying damages trust. First we lose the trust of others, then we lose the trust we may have had in ourselves. We can never quite reclaim our believability with others. We struggle to reclaim it even within ourselves. Lies also compound. One usually requires a collection of lies to follow, and soon the web of untruths is so complex that we cannot find our way out of the maze. Reclaiming the truth of the situation seems virtually impossible, over time.

A Parable

Once upon a time a woman decided to write a book. She wanted it to be a very good book and she wanted everyone to like it and think her and the book quite clever. She would have preferred wisdom but felt a bit unequal to the task. She was eager to write down all the clever things she knew. For many years, she had been very frustrated at all the people who wrote books and tucked little lies into them. "Not me, though!" she proclaimed.

Then she started to write the book. Every once in a while she would notice that she was cleverly writing about all manner of goofy and disturbing things that other people did. She kept mentioning that they did these things, sometimes with great enthusiasm. She meant well, of course, and was trying to tell everyone, in her book, about these goofy things. Some were so goofy that they had really hurt other people a great deal, so she got pretty serious about telling everyone about them.

Then one day, as she was writing about a goofy thing, she realized that this goofy thing was something she clearly did a lot herself. Well, that was pretty disturbing. She thought about that a few days. Then she went back and read everything she had written about goofy things. Little by little, she realized that everything she had written about other people doing goofy things was true of her. Everything!

Projection and Blaming

This may be the most popular of American sports. It is so rampant that it is difficult to describe it. At an uneven table, it enables me to avoid my contribution to an ineffective negotiation by laying blame and responsibility on the other party. I can simply show others the error of their ways. I can attack them, belittle them, discount them, accuse them, ridicule them, patronize them. I do these things, I like to think, because they need to be shown the error of their ways.

The nice thing about projection and blaming is that everyone else at an uneven table comes there with some human vulnerability, some fault, some limitation hanging out of their sleeve or even emblazoned on their sweatshirt. It isn't hard to find something flawed in others. It isn't even clever, actually. Then, when I find myself uncomfortable, all I need to do is quickly point to the flaw in another, deflecting attention from my own responsibility. I need not own my own limitations or failure to act. After it all: it was all their fault! As noted earlier, projection of the shadow is a particularly virulent version of this maneuver.

A Parable

Once upon a time, there was a person who was reading a book. In the book, the person read a parable. It was kind of a funny one about an author who found out that everything she was writing about other people was actually true of herself. The reader thought that this was pretty interesting, and wondered how that author could actually presume to write a book when she had all those faults. The reader didn't think much more about the parable. The reader was at least relieved that it was about the author, and other people, and, thank the heavens, not the reader.

Never Really Being There

This maneuver is more common than is at first apparent, but it has a certain subtlety to it that makes it harder to identify. I can actually go to the table to negotiate, discover it is uneven, withdraw, and just leave my mask, my false self, my public persona at the table. I can also simply behave myself and become compliant and passive. I can attend with only a small part of me there, or virtually none of me there.

Some people are so absent to themselves all the time that they don't even realize that they are doing this. The advantage of this state of affairs is that they can treat a negotiated agreement like a nice discussion without any outcomes. No agreement is ever achieved because there is really no one there to agree with or, for that matter, to disagree with. Such exchanges have a short-term relief potential and a long-term danger attached.

The most insidious impact of this approach is that persons using it may agree to all manner of destructive activities, even to themselves, and believe that since they didn't really consent, they are not responsible. They can convince themselves that in their hearts, they held firmly to the good and true, but that all the other people at the table were responsible because they participated. They can even convince others of their innocence, as if the refusal to act was a good in itself. When the refusal to act furthers a destructive outcome through silence, the impact of this approach becomes apparent. Hannah Arendt (1963) has amply demonstrated this in her analysis of Eichmann at Jerusalem.

actress

the only difference
between my sham
and common sham
is
i call it sham

i face the footlights
head-on:
i perform.

others
think it real,
but then,
others
call their sham
reality.

—pbk

Never Really Leaving

This maneuver is as effective as never really being there and often more effective. Here I can stay at the table and create a negotiation stalemate. I refuse to change, reach agreement, or move. I take no responsibility for the stalemate. I just stay. I may be quite good at showing why nothing will work, why no solution is viable. I may also simply silently brood, register modest signals of disapproval or dismay, yet take no action. Others may even be drawn into trying to elicit my approval, especially if I am holding some emotional hostages. Or I may simply sulk.

It is sometimes unclear why a person stays under these conditions. It has occurred to me, on occasion, that maybe they just don't have any other place to go. Here, at this table, uneven though it be, they exist. They can induce others to carry them, to keep cajoling and coaching them. They are the proverbial deadwood of an organization. Sometimes they can consume enormous amounts of the time and energy of others if this maneuver is not recognized for what it is. It is often passive aggression looking placid as a puddle. It is often deliberate helplessness posing as trust and involvement. Sometimes it is a maneuver for control because the efforts of all other participants are directed at evoking involvement or addressing the concerns of this person. This maneuver can effectively deter creative initiatives.

close

he had
only courage enough
for glancing blows
of intimacy,
delivered silently
in dark tunnels,
when least expected,
on his terms only.

over the years,
bruised,
she learned to
call it battery,
and so, finally,
she left.

—pbk

Harmful Partnerships and Deals

This maneuver has a dangerous dimension to it, and is one I often struggle with because I want to be able to trust without demanding the level of discrimination it requires. I can thus easily lock myself into an ineffective negotiating position or behavior because I have inadvertently or carelessly become part of a coalition based on the assumption of my powerlessness or my victimhood. Suddenly, I am called on to deliver on a partnership where I had failed to see at the outset the potential harms in the "deal."

Once the deal is cut, of course, I find myself without the mobility and fluidity I need to grow, change, and create. Yet I believe that I cannot break the deal without losing face or seeming to not hold to my part of the bargain. I can suddenly find myself trapped, with both alternatives seeming problematic and unsolvable.

A Story

I of course am writing this book as part of some larger life story. When I first began writing, I was working to keep the tuition funds flowing for my children. Happily they have earned their degrees as I complete this second edition. My "day job" for several of the intervening years involved negotiating the process of creating a doctoral program in nursing. I had done this once before, which helped some, but every new political process is a series of new lessons.

Part of my job was meeting with other professors from other disciplines to elicit their involvement and assistance. This was a stimulating exercise for me, and I enjoyed it. Some colleagues were remarkably helpful and responsive. Some operated with an unstated assumption that mirrors society's most negative assumptions about nurses: that we are pleasant but not particularly bright, that we are not scholars or thinkers, that we simply do what others tell us to do. Since I operate with a very extensive experiential knowledge of the error in these assumptions, I enjoyed these exchanges less but felt competent to address the issues.

To find out the status of the person I was speaking with, I usually introduced this concern early in our conversation. This led to a variety of responses. One exchange involved a colleague explaining to me his reasons for believing nursing scholarship did not meet his standards of rigor. He noted that nurses write their "opinions" and call this scholarship. I noted that philosophy was essentially the discussion of "opinions." He noted that nurses wrote opinions that did not cite large numbers of experts who would support what they were saying. I noted that originality was the most substantive and creative part of scholarship. We went on in this fashion for some time.

What I realized somewhere in this exchange was that this colleague did not believe my discipline had met his expectations, and that his help, which he generously offered to me numerous times, would only be given if I accepted the premise that nursing scholarship was defective and needed to be repaired, preferably using his measures of excellence. Had I consented to this help, I would have cut a deal with the assumption of my own powerlessness and my inadequacy as a given and would have participated in my own victimization.

An Exercise

The above discussion of manipulative maneuvers was of course not exhaustive. It was largely illustrative. Its purpose has been to give you as the reader a chance to review your own behaviors, habits, tendencies, and propensities. As is obvious, it could also help you to understand the behavior of others. If you like projection and blaming a great deal, this discussion can also be used destructively, to accuse other people of certain behaviors while ignoring your own. In the spirit of avoiding that kind of destructive nonsense, here's an exercise to help you focus on this list as one pertaining to you rather than to others. You will need the list of methods of maneuvering to do this exercise, so here it is:

I Won't and I Don't Because I Can't

Cynicism

Holding Emotional Hostages

Humoring the Fools

Emotional Numbing and Deadening

Some Lies Are Okay Because I Mean Well

Projection and Blaming

Never Really Being There

Never Really Leaving

Harmful Partnerships and Deals

Copy the methods of maneuvering. Make a list of them. Then study each of them for a while. Pretend you use all ten. It is of course possible that you have evolved well beyond the rest of the species and use none of them, or only one or two, but for purposes of this exercise, pretend you use all ten.

After you have studied them for a while, put the number one beside the one you like the best, a two beside the one you like second best, and on down to ten. This is a rank order. Now rank order them according to the one that irks you the most in others. Do this from one to ten. Now study these rankings. Any news here?

While you're trying to figure out the news in that rank-order exercise, here are some other thoughts to keep you on edge while you struggle with that question. As you can see, all of these maneuvers are based on emotional immaturity. Since these are emotional responses, they cannot be addressed with intellectual solutions or interventions. For those of you who hoped you could think them away, this is doubtless bad news of a sort. However, if you're carrying around some goofy emotional immaturities anyway, they can hardly be doing you any good, even when you're not at an uneven table, so why would you want to cling to them?

These maneuvers are emotional and thus require interventions of the heart. They are immaturities and thus require change and growth. They are personal in character and thus, while I may be able to change them in myself, I may not be able to even modestly influence them in others. Changing from behaviors that are expressions of emotional immaturity to other more productive and creative behaviors is an exercise of a type of power that is called personal agency. It is a type of power that stands in sharp contrast to that type of power called dominance power.

The good news is that personal agency power feels good. It also has many positive outcomes and is not limited to those that occur at an uneven table. It increases my sense of self-worth and is likely to dramatically improve the chances of a positive outcome when I negotiate at an uneven table. Thus, it has a good deal of promise but requires of me a commitment to emotional maturity. My ability to let go of these methods of maneuvering and to try new, more productive behaviors is actually the measure of my commitment to developing emotional maturity. Another way of looking at the same issue is to find out what kind of children show up at uneven tables.

12

Children at an Uneven Table

Two kinds of children show up at uneven tables, both manifesting common versions of emotional immaturity. The first is the omnipotent child, who must control the situation and prevail to feel safe, to sustain a sense of personal adequacy. This child says, "I know I am right and it has to be my way or it won't be at all." The second is the powerless child who believes that personal safety lies in the hands of others. This child has despaired of having self-agency or never wanted the responsibility for it in the first place. This child says, "I know I have no power to change anything, so others must do for me what I believe I cannot do for myself." Sometimes these children come in groups or partnerships of one kind or another.

It probably won't really surprise you to learn that neither child is capable of effective negotiation. Unfortunately, both children lurk somewhere in all of us and often become more apparent when the unevenness of the table becomes apparent. The omnipotent child, realizing that others are or seem to be powerless, begins to engage in controlling behaviors. The actions themselves may be benevolent, even protective, but they are designed to sustain the lack of personal agency and personal responsibility in the powerless. The omnipotent child uses this process to further substantiate the need to exercise dominant power, even arguing that the situation requires it.

The helpless child, realizing that others appear more powerful, can then drift into any of the manipulative maneuvers described above. The behaviors themselves may appear as benevolent as those of the omnipotent child. But they are designed to avoid personal agency and personal responsibility. They give one's autonomy to those exercising dominant power. The helpless child uses this process as further evidence of the persistence of victimization and the hopelessness of ever trying to exercise power.

Seeking to mature beyond the behaviors of these children asks a great deal of us, and we tend to want others to overlook the behaviors or to solve the problems our behaviors create. We may drift to cynicism, intellectualizing our way out of an honest confrontation with the issues, failing to see our involvement in furthering what are essentially constraints on our hearts and souls.

We don't want to stare at these two little kids too much. If we did, we might notice that both of them bring a very confined definition of their own self-interest to the table. The self-interest in either simplistic control or a refusal of simple self-responsibility are both narrow, shallow, and immediate agendas. What is perhaps less noticeable is that if you harbor one, you harbor the other. The omnipotent child has a hidden helplessness that is veiled with all that aggression; the helpless child has a hidden omnipotence that is veiled with all that manipulation. Both dimensions are always present; often, if one doesn't work, we try the other.

A Disclaimer

We haven't had a disclaimer yet! It's something new to keep you alert. Those of you who are thinking while you read this book have by now noticed that you keep picturing other people when I describe these behaviors. You may even have started writing a Christmas list of all the people who should read this book so they can see what jerks they can be. This demonstrates that your participation in the national sport of projection and blaming is alive and well. The shadow knows.

You may have also noticed that some of what I say seems to describe women and some of what I say seems to describe men, at least as you read it. Everything I'm describing I think of as merely human, but I think we live in a culture where we have so rigidly defined sex roles, and so forcefully tried to challenge this rigidity, that the gender dimension of what I describe in this book is central. More pointedly, conflict is always first of all an inner process and emerges when we feel a difference with another. The first way we all discover that we differ with others on a systematic basis is by reason of gender. Thus, it is our first model of difference and conflict.

As a result, much human conflict seems linked to gender. We even talk a good deal about "the war of the sexes." It's a pretty fundamental source of conflict in our culture. Thus, it will often emerge as an issue as your understanding of conflict increases. This is a common experience, and no doubt needs to be explored much more systematically. It is not, however, the focus of this book. It is a book I hope to write someday, but it is not the focus of this book.

This is said to acknowledge that this topic needs exploration, that its absence in this book creates a certain "missing piece" sensation occasionally, and that this can be confounding. It is also said to advise you that I agree, and want to try to write about all of that eventually, albeit not now. The utility of this book is that you can continue to read and study about uneven tables without trapping yourself in the assumptions about gender in our society. All humans end up at uneven tables, all humans try to find ways to cope with this fact, and all humans could use some help in the coping. That there are structured and reinforced ways for men and women to cope is true, but knowing this is not essential to your either understanding or addressing an uneven table.

This disclaimer is provided to put the question to bed, for the time being, acknowledging the need to return to it at a later date.

An Exercise

Get your journal out again. Go back to your rank-ordered list of manipulative maneuvers. Beside each one, indicate whether you think men or women use this one more. Now compare this to the rank of which ones you prefer, of which ones irk you the most. This is pretty interesting stuff, isn't it?!

Families at an Uneven Table

Once you're willing to have your children at an uneven table, it is only a matter of moments before you discover that you have families at the table. I made the disclaimer above for that reason. The children at the table are our unresolved immaturities, and once they show up, we catapult ourselves backward to our early days and go in search of Mom and Dad, or those who served in their place. To our chagrin, we may not find them there, or if we do, they may not be doing their job as we expect them to do, but the search will occur.

Our culture has certain assumptions about a family system. We spend a good deal of time trying to fix, honor, save, proclaim, salvage, perpetuate, or lament the American family. These assumptions are made manifest in everyone's childhood, with varying degrees of congruence with the messages that surround any given family about the nature of being a family. We learn these as we switch from pureed food to solids, and the lumps can be about equally difficult to manage. Over time, these images get reinforced, and we live by them, even trying to recreate or improve on them as adults.

Family systems are thus one of the first examples we have of how to negotiate at an uneven table. In our culture, omnipotent and helpless children negotiate with parents and siblings as best they can, in both cases assuming a degree of unevenness. In our culture, this unevenness is viewed as a given, with the adults in charge of dominant power. Sibling order and sibling rivalry are studied as meaningful dynamics, and we all nod and concur without much conscious attention to the ways these things shape our behavior at uneven tables.

If we are unaware of this process, we can quickly drift to perceiving the uneven table as "a lot like home, when I was a kid" and not even know we are doing this. Suddenly, someone at the table is dad, someone else is mom, someone else a big brother or a little sister. We begin to negotiate from this position and expect others to adapt. We act as we have always acted, in a compulsion of repetition, and then wonder why "people always react to me that way."

We hold these compulsive behaviors dear in part because they are so primal; we've used them from birth and we deeply want them to work, to evoke a response. We may have actually had some fairly unwanted responses, but we learned early that this is how to get involved in the family system and be a member. We often protect these behaviors from honest scrutiny. We may even think such scrutiny is disloyal and could create a threat to our base of support—our fundamental love relationships—our family. We indeed may have actively continued to use these behaviors in our family systems and never even considered that alternatives were available or held more potential than the ones we're using.

This situation is further complicated by the fact that we may then elect, as adults, to design an "instant replay" of our family of origin, further strengthening our commitment to the behaviors. We repeat these relationships, sustain them, and teach them to the next generation. This increases our investment in getting them to work sort of exponentially. We don't really want to investigate them because to do so is to actually question both our earliest and our current base of support. We need all this to be right the way it is; we are reluctant to discover its limits.

While all of this role playing may seem to decrease anxiety, and provides at least the secondary comfort of familiarity, it leaves us playing out roles and scripts that are more characteristic of an immature and unconscious child than those of an adult. We are thus not only framed more by societal expectations than our own intrinsic self, but participate in furthering the claims such structures make on others. This is a virtual truism demonstrated in disturbing processes such as child abuse and other acts of violence. We are, however, reluctant to admit that our own little generational patterns can be equally problematic and require equal scrutiny and exposure. Under such conditions, self-agency is at best an illusion.

One of the most troublesome outcomes of this process is the intermixing of love with dominant power, of a sense of self-adequacy with dynamics around dominant power. We find ourselves behaving as children and claiming we are engaged in adult discourse. We then feel a need to defend this charade, since our sense of self-worth is inextricably linked up with sustaining these roles and scripts. It is very difficult to put these factors into some detached and honest self-appraisal.

———————

A Story

I am fortunate in regard to this dynamic. I am from a large family. When I go to an uneven table, if I want to be unconscious and immature, I can assign a large number of roles to people at the table before I run out of family members. I have an older sister, an older brother, two younger sisters, and three younger brothers. This gives me lots of opportunities to play roles I learned as a child.

One of my sisters died when I was ten. She was almost seven at the time, and her death had an enormous impact on me. Among other things, I was stunned by the fragility of the human, and began to think of younger sisters and brothers as persons who were vulnerable, who indeed could die. I concluded that they needed protection. As a result, at most uneven tables, I find these vulnerable others and want to protect them with a frenzy.

It has taken me a long time to modify this behavior, and it still beckons me on a regular basis. I know intellectually that to further another person's self-agency is a wiser and more humane gesture, but it is easy for me to bypass that challenge and slide into protection. I know it is irrational to try to save others, especially if they do not elect to take self-responsibility, but I still drift toward advocacy on their behalf. If others at the table seem reluctant to honor this vulnerability and advocacy, I get irked and become convinced that in their hearts they are murderous villains. I know that this is nonsense, but I learned the lesson early, and it still can capture me emotionally and behaviorally.

It is my hope that everyone who was totally exasperated with me over the last thirty years when I behaved this way is reading this and saying, "Oh, now I get it!" and engaging in profound acts of compassion and forgiveness. The fact is, such compulsions and repetitions become our "signature," our public persona, our style of operation. They become so familiar and commonplace that we even call them human nature, which they are not. We like to think the habits of mind and heart that framed our youth are fixed entities that cannot be changed. But they are merely an image of today's evolutionary moment, both for each of us as individuals and for humans as a collective. Those most normalized by a culture become the highest point on the normal curve of human evolution. As is obvious, however, this highest point can move, has moved, and indeed, if we continue to grow and evolve, inevitably will move.

———————

13

Evolution at an Uneven Table

Evolution is not necessarily a goal during the negotiation of a conflict, even though it obviously could be. What often seems more common is the obverse: that success is framed as freedom from the call to evolve, to change, to grow. We may even feel we are successful in a negotiation precisely because we do not have to grow. This is kind of a weird belief system, but it does show up with a great deal of regularity.

We often embrace the automatic simple solution to a complex problem in an effort to stave off the more demanding solution. We think we can silence or ignore the call to evolve, as if ignoring the call to eat or walk would have no effect over time. We bring our histories, our prides, our fears, our insecurities, and our need to prevail into our negotiations and present these with greater vigor and clarity than we bring our search for the evolutionary opportunity, the chance to change and grow. We think somehow that to admit growth is to imply that yesterday, less evolved, we were defective. Honoring our own organic growing and evolving comes to us as a struggle, not a liberation.

This seems to be true to some degree of most humans, and not surprisingly havoc emerges quite predictably. We should expect nothing else when a negotiation is focused on the lowest common denominator of what it means to be human. If we assume that the negotiation will further the immaturities and repetition compulsions of the participants, rather than giving them an opportunity to evolve beyond these fixations, the outcome is quite predictable.

We then seek the path of least resistance. We pursue the morally expedient outcome. We suppress our covert despair and hopelessness. We assume the worst in other participants. We honor the insistent voice of cynicism. We get what we expect!

Ultimately, we are asking ourselves to be less than we are and less than we can become. This is poignantly true of many uneven tables, whether we see ourselves as dominant or subordinate, privileged or disadvantaged, superior or inferior. Either way, we have an opportunity to evolve or fixate, to diminish or enlarge ourselves, to move toward that which is best about being human or toward more poverty of mind and soul. If we actively embrace such poverty of mind and soul, we should not be surprised that it lurks in our lives with such tenacity.

_____

An Exercise

Remember the exercise at the beginning of this part of the book, before you bravely slogged your way through all the ways of being a traditionalist at an uneven table? I asked you to write down the five ways you most commonly use manipulation with others. I told you we would revisit this list. The time is now.

Flip back through your journal and see if you can locate the list. If you can't, that is the first thing you can learn from this exercise. If you find the list, study it for a while. See how much you would like to keep it just as it is, how you might like to change it, how you feel about it. This may turn out to be the best indicator you've had thus far concerning your basic willingness to evolve. Change is so nice in theory, so welcome when someone else changes for the better, evolves. Unfortunately, the only evolution you and I personally control, however, is our own. The first step involves getting honest with ourselves about our interest in change. We make choices.

_____

Evolving Beyond Traditional Approaches to an Uneven Table

We all have the option to choose to evolve beyond these traditional approaches to an uneven table. It is not critical which roles we tend to play most frequently at such tables. The issue is more the honest recognition of the limited utility of all these roles, and the willingness to consider that something more satisfying, gratifying, and self-fulfilling is available. To make this choice, however, seems to me to elect the road "less traveled." As Robert Frost (1969) notes, this will make all the difference, however, and we need to attend to that fact.

Taking a new road may increase our sense of aloneness. In some cases, we may actually be alone, "all-one" in ourselves. We may even have to cut a new trail where none now exists. We may find such a challenge risky, lonely, or fatiguing. We need to reflect on the implications of such a choice, and determine the degree to which this alternative appeals to us.

An Exercise

Return once more to the list of ten manipulative maneuvers. Take your top three favorites. List them. Now, write two or three brief examples of where you most like to use these, such as "my wife always responds to this one well" or "this works at conferences most of the time." Now imagine yourself in these situations. Imagine that you have promised yourself to never use these behaviors again. This is merely imagining. For the record, they don't go away from such omnipotent promises . . . they just get suppressed or come in with new costumes.

Now, how do you feel about not having these handy little maneuvers available? Do you miss them already? Does it make you feel kind of anxious to be in these situations without the maneuvers to fall back on? Can you even imagine an alternative? Will people think something awful has happened to you if you quit using these maneuvers? What will you do about that?

As this exercise indicates, entertaining the notion of giving up our traditional approaches to an uneven table evokes a whole list of insistent questions that will not be subdued. The following list is merely exemplitive, but begins to make reflective consideration more of a reality: Do I want to evolve or not? What will it cost me? Am I ready? Why? How ready? Where am I not ready yet? Why? Can I absent myself from the challenge since I believe I have just proven that I'm not ready? How much can I absent myself? Do I want to get ready? How much? How will I go about it? Am I willing to pay the price? What is the price? Is it too much? Why? Can I be compassionate with myself and others as I seek answers to these questions? Do I ask an evolution of others that I am not yet ready to embrace myself? Do I claim others should evolve but absolve myself? Why? Do I want conflict to be diminished or resolved in my life without my involvement? Why? What do I want to do about all of this?

The easier solution, that of sustaining immaturities and repetition compulsions, beckons us abruptly. Despite the embarrassment of self-diminishment, we may elect to sustain the traditional approaches, even though we know clearly that these solve nothing and in fact do damage by sustaining conflict. Honestly feeling the seduction of these traditional approaches is important. Struggling with our fondness for them is worth discovering. It may even make us more compassionate with all the folks who, having asked the questions listed above, decided that for them, tradition will prevail.

New Pathways

Others of us may decide to travel a different road. In the process, we will encounter adventures, rewards, life-expanding challenges, and growth opportunities. We always have to pay a price for such things, of course, and the price may prove to be a high one. But life, any way we live it, has a price. If this is the case, why not a price that brings into our lives these more fulfilling options?

healing the caverns of the heart

i have no means of divining all
the endless pathways in this heart,
no light source illumines silken crevices,
or whole vast plains of patterning
in darkling times; space grows, flows
cavernous, stretching rigid bands and
comfort boundaries. i cannot see.
worse still, i cannot now retreat,
and looking back, i'm startled
to discover simple platitudes and
sentimental wanderings still light seduction
themes: they lilt some siren ditty to
the blinded soul, groping along the
endless, infirm, unfirm walls of
this relentless maze. as a child i
dreamed a dream of fire beyond
proportions, and now, burned empty,
i seek the child among the ashen waste:
to give advice, cajole, draw her back
from the edge where clarity eludes.
i would not want to have engaged my
life among the cushions of the safety
zone, and envy no one there, really,
in the end, but think on all the
reasons why the one who pays no price
may pay the endless every price there is.
i harbor neither lucid, nor later rancid,
nor mere wan regrets

> *—pbk*

Actually, though we may seem alone at an uneven table when we pursue a new approach to the challenge, and take our leave of traditional approaches, we are in one sense never really alone. We discover that those who have gone before us can give us some guide-lines, that those who are struggling toward the same goal can be our companions on the journey. We can support, sustain, encourage, and congratulate one another. We need not do this alone. It is actu-ally kind of fun to be with the people on the road less traveled. They are usually much more interesting than the people repeating all the traditional approaches to unevenness. They are creative and alive. And they are always giving us new opportunities to try new pathways with them.

14

Imagining New Approaches to an Uneven Table

We can choose to let go of traditional approaches to an uneven table, or at least consider the possibility. Several decision points emerge immediately. These need to be attended to early in the process and become critical if we feel "forced" to be at an uneven table. In reality, we are never forced to be there, since there are a variety of ways of not being there, and there are really no forces putting us there. But we may choose to be there for some reason so compelling that not being there seems impossible. What we may discover is that we are not so much forced to be there as we are unwilling to accept the consequences of not being there. It is useful to make this distinction.

Beyond the decision points, there are a series of outcomes that require a reframing of reality. This too can be challenging, since the reality presented may seem quite incongruent with the reframing we hope to achieve. Both the decision points and the reframing process require concerted effort and focused attention.

Decision Points

Several decisions have to be made in approaching an uneven table. We need to make as careful an appraisal of the situation as possible, which can best be achieved by answering a series of questions about this particular uneven table. The meanings we give to these questions are unveiled as we grapple with the questions themselves.

Why am I going to this table? What do I hope to achieve? What am I willing to do to achieve this? If we have motives that contradict the goal of resolving the conflict or creatively participating in the negotiation, we are already ill-equipped to deal with the table's unevenness. If we want to achieve our goals through a loss of personal humanity or integrity, we are even more at risk. We may find we want to demand moral stature in others without demanding moral behavior of ourselves, or we may want to protect our resistive blind spots, or we may want to continue to lie to ourselves while demanding honesty and self-confrontation from others.

What are the rules at the table? Do I accept them? Can I change them? If I find I don't like the rules, do I lie and pretend I accept them? Do I introduce my alternatives honestly? If they are rejected, what do I do next? Do I have a plan for dealing with this eventuality? We cannot seek alternatives if we begin the negotiation with deception. If the rules cannot be changed and I do not accept them, staying at the table creates new conflicts. It taints the entire process.

What is being negotiated at the table, overtly and covertly? If the overt issue is dominance or control, and I am to be the one controlled, why am I at the table? What are we negotiating for? If the covert issue is dominance or control, will it be made overt? By whom? Knowing the precise nature of the power concerns at the table is helpful. This may take some "homework," but the preparation time is ultimately valuable in enabling clarity of judgment.

Is the dominance or control being negotiated around symbols of dominance: fame, money, social status, educational credentials, vanities, beauty, self-aggrandizement? How important are these issues to me? Do they attract me? Am I willing to enhance them in others? How? Why? In what manner? Enhancing these qualities in others may not have a direct impact on me, but could do harms to others at the table. If I seem to endorse these qualities, then I may become party to the harms that emerge.

Are there issues I consider important that need to be negotiated? Can they be negotiated? Will they be negotiated, or is this merely a formality? Will these issues be resolved on the basis of dominance? Will this be acceptable to me? To what extent could I be asked to compromise my personal integrity? Am I willing to pay this price? Unless these issues are addressed, I may simply drift to the table because the issues are important to me without realizing what other factors can shape the outcomes.

What risks do I take? What price must I pay? Are these worth it to me? Why? Risks for their own sake make little sense and squander time, energy, and effort. Knowing the price that could be paid and the dangers inherent in the price are important issues to face before the fact, not after I get there and find I have to make a decision under duress.

Who else will be at the table? Do any of the other participants seek the same goals as I do? Where and when are they likely to pursue another course of action? Does all this matter to me? How much? Why? If I find that the others at the table are likely to support or oppose my efforts to be at the table in a nontraditional way, what may emerge from the process can have a substantive impact on me. Assessing this beforehand can be useful and informative.

What do I think I'm unable to handle? How might I fail? Am I representing others who count on me to succeed? How do I experience this obligation or responsibility? Are the losses I could experience worth the risk? Are they worth the gains? In what ways am I too ineffective to be at the table under these conditions? Do I anticipate harming myself or others? Should I do this? These questions are harder to answer, but for that reason more compelling. Harms that could emerge are often a key indicator about the actual nature of an uneven table. If these harms will accrue to others beyond myself, this adds an additional burden to the decision.

What processes will be attempted? Can I handle these? If so, why? If not, why not? Should someone other than me be sitting at this table? Will they? How could I help them if they would? These questions get to the more substantive issues that emerge at an uneven table and to the methods used to sustain inequity. They thus provide a more robust picture of the challenge and provide a better information base for informed decision making.

A Story

An example here might help. It also might keep you from drowning in a list of tough questions. I once faced exactly this kind of challenge, and while I had already made a decision to present myself at the table as someone on a new path rather than one wedded to traditional behaviors, I think it demonstrates nicely the scope and nature of the questions and what they might reveal.

I was invited to participate in a two-day decision process aimed at creating a board of directors that would guide a health care center whose mission was to improve access to health care for underserved populations. I was invited as the dean of a large university-based school of nursing. I was ostensibly invited to represent the interests of nursing. I was interested in crafting a center that would meet the community's health care needs and that would allow caregivers to work together rather than competitively.

Many factors were weighed in my decision, however. I very much wanted to have nursing well represented in this process, and on the board of directors. For many years, in nearly every major health enterprise, nurses have been systematically excluded from serving on boards of directors, despite the fact that they are the largest group of health care providers. In hospitals, they are always the largest employee group. They do a great deal to further the image and success of the hospital yet are rarely considered for board positions. Physicians, in contrast, almost always have representatives on the board even though often they are not employed by the hospital and may have a lesser stake in hospital outcomes because they have greater mobility. This chronic injustice was and is a source of ongoing irritation for me, since the board often makes decisions that have a very deleterious effect on nurses. The frustration I had felt about this over the years led to a more intense stubbornness than might be effective or useful. I wasn't sure I could get beyond it to larger issues.

I also felt strongly that the interests of minority communities should be a major consideration in staffing the board. They had clearly communicated that they needed an assurance that the health care would be community based and culturally responsive. I wanted to help create the change needed to make that happen and felt that having a "white" person involved would be of some use or value.

The decision process, however, was primarily controlled by the local school of medicine, since it had been awarded the money that made the center possible. While school representatives expressed awareness of and interest in my goals, I had no assurance that these would be honored. If they were not, the invitation to be coopted by the medical school's contrasting goals could emerge. In addition, I believed that since the medical school had legal responsibility for the funds, school officials were entitled to have some degree of control in board decisions. Some members of the community hoped they would have little or no input.

Two outside consultants were called in for these two days, and in meeting with them I asked the questions about process that I needed answers to in order to assure myself that I did trust and respect the competence of the consultants. This helped considerably. I was candid with the two consultants and pointed out what I saw as the problems confronting me. They did not promise to solve them, and did not discredit my goals. They thus seemed both realistic and honest to me. This helped move me closer to the table.

While the overt issue at the table was board composition, the covert agenda was control. Had the representatives from the medical school sought all the control, I would not have gone to the table. While some people who expressed the views of the medical school wanted complete control, others were willing to seek a balance between board members who represented the medical school's interests and board members who represented other health professions and community interests. This signaled that not all the negotiations would be around historic dominant control issues, though some would be.

I evaluated who might better represent my views. Since I had been involved in this process for some time, I was an established participant. I would find the focus on control tedious, since it was not my major concern, but I would have to accept this. I would find few opportunities to raise issues of more importance to me, which could make me impatient and frustrated. I needed to face this. While I had enough experience to know that many views at the table make for a richer outcome, and hence heterogeneity at the table was my goal, the effort to represent nursing would probably be interpreted not as my effort to ensure that heterogeneity but merely as self-interest.

While members of other health professions would be present, these participants would represent other institutions with their own nursing programs. I expected that these participants would only support nursing goals if they included or favored their institution. The issue of nursing in decision-making processes was not a central agenda for these persons. Indeed, the fact that they were representing other groups while nursing had a representative was a source of discontent for some. These players, like everyone else, struggled with the issue of control as the central agenda, and it would shape most of their activity at the table.

Perhaps the most complex dimension for me was the fact that I was a white woman at the table. I could understand and negotiate with the white physicians who were worried about adequate medical school control. I understood their worldview, though they did not understand mine, nor were they willing to actively represent it. I could understand and negotiate with the members of the community who were worried about adequate community control. I even shared this agenda with them, though less directly than my concern about nursing. My concern about nursing was not one that they actively represented. The assumption that since I was a white woman I would have my interests represented by white men was also present, although unstated. The fact that I was a white woman led to the assumption by some participants that I would take the view of white men present and adopt it as my own. Indeed, it was assumed that the women of color would support the men of color present. Some assumed, too, that since I was a nurse, I would support medicine; others assumed that since I was a nurse, I would oppose medicine.

These things I could anticipate, and they indeed happened as described. The discontent my seeming ethnic nonpartisanship created became one of the most challenging outcomes. The price of failing to uphold "white" or established medicine's interests by supporting the community representatives involved a cost, and asked more, retrospectively, than I expected I would have to pay. Since I was a dean at the time, making sure that this did not have an adverse impact on my school was an added concern. The well-being of nursing was furthered, but not as clearly as I had hoped. I worried that I might not have represented my nursing colleagues as well as I might have had I been more partisan. All of these issues and others went into the appraisal of this situation and made the decision to go to this very uneven table a difficult one. I did go, and did not regret it, but the complexity of this table, with a group of over twenty people, gives a useful window on the importance of these questions. The issues I identified here actually only make up a partial list of issues at this table.

Moral Dilemmas

What these questions and the emergent answers tend to unearth are actually moral dilemmas, quandaries that ask whether this is the table to sit at or not, and why. There are many things in my life that are more vital, profound, compelling, and creative than power and control. I am more deeply and lastingly touched and moved by love, compassion, innovation, bliss, beauty, justice, and courage. If none of these are at a table, I need to continually ask myself why I am there. I need to determine if this table is worth my time and energy.

Many tables invite me because they promise to deliver something, or at least imply the possibility. I need to know if they really can deliver, and how. If the promise is justice, or voice, or parity, or influence, and these do not emerge, I need to know why. I also need to know exactly what price being at a table that fails to deliver these really exacts. Beyond the simple failure to deliver is the fact that I have given over my time and effort to an enterprise that could not honor my investments. The other costs of being at an uneven table are high enough; this just adds insult to injury.

I am invited to some tables because my job or church or family says I must be there or something will happen to me. I need to look at this closely and see if it is true. What are the effects of being present and how do these relate to the effects of not being present? Does my presence suggest that I let myself be coerced into being at tables? Would my absence send a more constructive message?

I am invited to some tables to give the appearance of justice or fairness. I am a token. Then I must ask if my presence involves cooptation. I also need to ask if I am participating to prove myself better than or more responsive than other "powerless people" who have refused to come to the table. I may also come to provide myself with an arena where I can act out my anger at those I feel have oppressed and victimized me. I may not want to really solve the conflicts. I may want to keep them going for the pleasure of punishing the oppressors. I need to really know why I am there, and if any good can come of it.

If I know that I have been invited as a concession, I need to know that there may be a large, albeit covert price to pay for that concession. I need to ascertain what that price will be and determine if the price is worth it to me or to others. I need to determine if I can or will pay the price. I need to know what, if any, threats to my personal integrity will emerge, or whether my participation will later be viewed merely as complicity, endorsement, and acceptance of outcomes I cannot support. I need to clearly differentiate between ends and means. I need to know if those setting the table believe the ends justify the means, and the degree to which they expect me to concur with this viewpoint which is unacceptable to me.

These are not easy issues, and they ask a great deal of a person considering participating at an uneven table. This is perhaps why so many people give up or never show up. The process of moral decision making in these cases can take a disproportionate amount of time and energy, since the person approaching an uneven table knowingly faces different moral dilemmas than those persons who fail to see or understand that the table is uneven, and that this unevenness will make all the difference.

It perhaps merits comment that it is easy to become captured by dismay, pouting, or resentment that one must engage in this process. I know that this happens to me sometimes. It seems unfair that I have to go through all these machinations just to try to negotiate for something that I think is intrinsically a good thing. It also seems unfair that those with disproportionate dominant power and control seem to be exempted from this process. Over time, however, I have learned to think of myself as the more fortunate person, since both the learning and the personal enrichment I have gained are substantive and valuable to me in day-to-day living. I have learned over time to think of those engaged in unconscious or unthinking injustice as disadvantaged, and this has led to a greater willingness to do my homework, and to do so with less petulance. It has also helped me realize that change in these structures will of necessity come from those who are disadvantaged rather than those with dominant power. Paulo Freire (1997) has done a superb job of providing an in-depth analysis of this virtual truism.

Clarifying My Place at the Table

The appraisal of the potential uneven table concludes with a set of decisions. If, based on the answers to the questions I've explored, I decide to go to the table, I then take the time to clarify for myself, sort of in summary, my own personal positions, philosophies, aims, intents, limits, and interests. This set of clarifications emerges somewhat as a process.

I need to know my own frame on reality, and very specifically on the conflicts or potential conflicts stemming from the fact that the table is uneven. I need to be ready and willing to articulate all of these things while at the table, and to do so clearly and objectively. I must also be ready to try to identify distortions in my sense of reality that emerge while I am at the table.

I then need to clarify the nature of the conflict at hand in light of these other considerations. Often this process makes it possible for me to see the conflict in a new light, or many new lights, to understand it better and see the multiplicity of dimensions it includes. This keeps the conflict light in my mind and heart, because I know it is complex, like human living and learning, and yet simple, like human living and learning.

This moves me to the next phase of clarification that involves identifying the skills, abilities, and attitudes I need to sit at this particular table in a "new" way, in a manner that moves me and the negotiation beyond the traditional approaches to an uneven table. I also need to face the fact that what are described as viable options for me by experts in conflict negotiations simply may not fit, since my perspective is not congruent with the one guiding the experts.

Since I know I am choosing to behave in ways that contradict norms, I then take time to carefully identify, to the best of my ability, my own limits, vulnerabilities, incapacities, undeveloped potentials, information gaps, biases, faults, and weaknesses. I have to conclude this process with the recognition that I probably have some important blindnesses still lurking somewhere, but that I can at least take responsibility for the ones I've found and faced. This is kind of a jittery process for me, but I think it's essential. If nothing else, when someone tries to discredit me by telling me about one of my limitations, I don't need to get defensive. We may even come up with the same stunning insight into my imperfection.

The final phase in this process of preparing myself involves clarifying my commitment to engagement at the table. I seek to ground myself in myself, to commit to self-responsibility based on self-awareness. I always posit to myself the possibility that I may have to sustain these alone, that there indeed may be no other person at the table prepared to be "with me." Being "all one" in oneself becomes critical, because I might actually be alone, and I need to be prepared for that potentiality. As unwelcome as the realization may be, I do ask myself to face the fact that no one else may elect to go on the path I choose to take.

The Afterflow Afterglow

*We shall win and perish. We shall
last beyond these fatalistic shadows
of our acrid disconnections. We shall
come stumbling as latter day saints,
finding lights beyond a christmas or
the milky way, energetic enveloping;
aflame beyond our limited imaginings.
Dimensions we're deserted or denied,
defiled with murmured homicides of
fear or pride or drive; frights on
journeys twined and ivied, burning
clear, uncluttering; now touchable
to everything alive: we come by only
opening to the coming. We shall be
more than only we create because we
are receiving, and have danced the
ever nurturing sensuous dance.*

—pbk

Anticipating Mystery

These preparations for seating oneself at an uneven table, as helpful
as they have proven to be for me, do not exhaust the possibilities of
what can emerge, and they cannot be pursued in that spirit. One
must be ready for human nature and mystery to play roles not yet
imagined. In my experience, one must be ready for both the unexpected betrayal or attack and the unexpected miracle. One must be
willing to accept and pay the price for the first, and embrace and
celebrate the second. This is easy to write, but staying my course
under attack or betrayal is very difficult for me, and I often have to
fight to stay in my own place and not drift back to the more traditional path. The miracle can be equally disorienting on occasion,
but for different reasons. I usually want to take the day off, dance in
the streets, raise a cup, the usual response to miracles. This sponta-

neous show of enthusiasm may deter the process rather than furthering it, however. I try to never neglect my congratulations, though I try to save them until after the process. They are no less sweet simply because of the delay. Sometimes they are sweeter.

The willingness to see, honor, attend to, and be prepared for both eventualities positions me in a way that enables me to honor the freedoms of others and the infinite potential of the human spirit, which always exceeds our cynical appraisal of it. It is perhaps significant in this regard that I rarely have a day where I don't get to celebrate at least one wonderful example of human courage or compassion. These events always move me, and I enjoy the pleasure they provide. That our daily news includes few, if any, of these events is more a commentary on our fixation on negativity as a culture than on what is really newsworthy. It always seems sort of shameful to me that we think these manifestations of human splendor are not of interest, and present them, when reported, in a sentimental and maudlin fashion, as if they were anachronisms. This says more about the soul of the media than it says of the events.

It has become acceptable to mask our betrayals and our splendor in this country. It is considered temperate, in good taste, even refined. The blunting of human sensibility, on the one hand, and the trivializing of mystery, on the other, are assaults on the human spirit. We wear many masks to cover both eventualities. The culture does not help us much in preparing ourselves for this dimension of an uneven table. Whenever you're on your own, though, remember that you get to write the rules of the game!

Reframing Reality in Approaching an Uneven Table

The recent enrichments in the philosophy of science, and in many other disciplines, have helped us see more clearly that the definitions of reality with which we operate, both as a species and individually, are largely a matter of social construction. The history of science is actually the history of creating new social constructions. Thus, our frame on reality becomes a critical dimension in our approach to an uneven table. This seems like a good time to provide a little summary report on the process of reframing reality that this book invites you to try.

All negotiation tables are uneven to some degree. Participants in the negotiation, including the negotiators, may deny, ignore, distort, or suppress this fact to some degree. If the evenness is denied, ignored, distorted, or suppressed, it exacerbates the conflict and intensifies the unevenness. Thus, both are sustained. Such sustaining actually contradicts the purported intent of conflict resolution, and thus must be constructively addressed.

There are traditional ways of responding to unevenness. They are actually models of how to sustain a conflict, at least covertly, by denying, ignoring, distorting, or suppressing the "reality" of unevenness. These are largely manipulative and sustain and reinforce the emotional immaturity of the participants. They are harmful.

If we wish to address the unevenness of a given table, and to do so constructively, this option exists. We must then introduce alternatives to the traditional responses to an uneven table. We're proposing, in essence, to construct new social realities. This includes not only the responses we make but the focus of the negotiation beyond issues of power and dominance. The construction of new social realities, in this context, essentially proposes new ways of being at an uneven table.

The next section of this book introduces you to those ways of being at an uneven table. It's about time, isn't it? You've been very gracious about reading this section. It's a tough one! All that self-confrontation. I think one last story is in order. This seems at first not to be directly about the book, but then, maybe it is. It can be used in the same fashion as the football story. That story introduced you to the spirit of my younger daughter; this one introduces you to the spirit of my older daughter. I know who my teachers are.

A Story

For my fiftieth birthday, my older daughter took me out to eat. It was an easy and relaxed experience, and I spent much of the time marveling at the mystery and wonder of this human I once knew only as abdominal kicking and squirming. She was twenty-two, and we were sharing stories of our recent histories.

Tricia had graduated from college nine months earlier and had decided to take two years to "live life," "become independent," "learn the value of a dollar," and other equally impressive goals before pursuing the next phase of her preparation for a career as a physician. She was full of wonderful stories. She had been a member of the Yale Women's Crew for her four years of college, a fact I report with obvious pride, and had since taken a job developing and coaching a youth rowing club.

We recalled together her phone call to me earlier in her experience with this club. She had two male assistant coaches. One of them, in visiting with one of the young men who was a member of the club and with his parents, had a conversation about who should coach the club. This assistant reported back to Tricia, somewhat casually, that they had all concurred that it might be better if one of the guys coached and Tricia could be the assistant.

Tricia had called me sputtering and fuming, "Is this not so sexist!" said in about twelve different ways. I tried to comfort her and point out that sexism on the job was often more tedious and trying. I was saddened for her but not surprised. She was offended, insulted, appalled. She kept repeating her concern as if my reaction didn't equal the nature of the crime.

In recounting this event, she said that she had actually often thought, while growing up, that I made too big a deal about sexism. She had never shared this, and indeed was more muted in her concern than I during those years. After this event, she told me, she began to say to herself, "Boy, my mom sure is calm and collected about sexism; how could she stand it all those years!" We laughed.

Turning serious, I told her then that I actually was saddened by the call, that I felt I had spent most of my career trying to create the conditions that would diminish injustice based on gender. I said I was saddened that I had seemed to make such a small dent in the problem. I had hoped to give her and her sister a bit better world to live their lives in. Some days, it seemed that so little change had been achieved.

"You have it all wrong, Mom," she responded. "Look at it this way. It took me twenty-two years to find out about it. All those other years I got to live my life without having to deal with it. That's a lot!"

Part Three

Constructive Ways of Being
at an Uneven Table

15

The Shift to New Ways of Being

This section of the book addresses the topic that probably led you to start reading this book: Are there some ways of being at an uneven table that I can learn about and benefit from? What are they? I realize that you might hope that I will now write the recipe, but as I noted at the beginning, that is not my intention. The ways of being discussed in this book are more of a gestalt. Thus, predictably, I want to start the description of these ways of being with a further perusal of context, the environment within which I believe one can best understand and experience these ways of being.

An Initial Shift in Reality: Ways of Being

What is a "way of being," anyway? I think the term sounds a bit odd, too, but I am trying to communicate something often ignored in our culture. In the United States, our social constructions usually try to give us access to new skills and abilities as if they were instant panaceas that one simply donned like new clothing. It is almost as if we think we can best create a new reality the way we create a costume: one white cotton sweater of openness, one dark cocoa pair of creativity pants, one pair of taupe suede loafers of sincerity, and one tasteful paisley decorative tie of integrity. New costume, new look; I must be living in a new reality! I have to admit the model has some appeal to me, and may explain my fascination at some subliminal level with mail-order catalogues. I fear it is much more demanding than that, however.

Ways of being, as I mean them here, refer to the manner, method, or approach with which one chooses to manifest his or her presence at an uneven table. It focuses on the "how" rather than the "what" of the situation.

If I want to create alternate or new realities, I need to go beyond the costuming approach to new experiences. Indeed, of their very nature, they cannot be dealt with in a costuming fashion, and to do so is to assure failure. Ignoring this fact, I run the risk of finding myself at an uneven table with others noting that the emperor's new clothes are fairly diaphanous. If the ways of being described here are treated as if they were simple skills to wear like Halloween costumes, masks and all, this would merely introduce new levels and versions of manipulation.

The human spirit thrives organically, not through manipulation, even though we become so confused sometimes that we are willing to manipulate our own hearts and souls. Because manipulation is ultimately a form of coercion and deceit, it serves no constructive purpose.

These ways of being, which propose to introduce alternate realities that will enable you to more constructively be at an uneven table, are also not presented as a simple checklist. They describe a field of action rather than a sequence of events or skills or abilities. Our culture likes easy and quick answers. I know this. I am not giving our culture what it likes here. I am doing this in a spirit of honesty, not insensitivity. It is deliberate.

Conflict is complex, inequity is complex, negotiation is complex. Constructively addressing these realities is inherently complex. Human growth is multidimensional. There are no easy answers. The certain thing one can know about an easy answer to a complex problem is that it is wrong.

These ways of being are also not discrete. This is not a taxonomy of parts or components. The ways of being interact, overlap, potentiate one another. It might be better to imagine them as the instruments in an orchestra. If all these instruments come together to express a beautiful theme by "playing their part," with you as the conductor, lovely music becomes possible. It is not assured, but the possibilities are at least entertained and given some hopeful attention. They are not static in nature; they are more catalysts than achievable goals. They are human potentials waiting for your knowing, deciding, and acting. They are all in your best interest, but they also ask something of you in the way a symphony score asks something of you.

All of these ways of being can be challenging and difficult to develop in oneself. They call forth compassion, both for oneself and for others. They require compassion, both for oneself and for others. They will never be fully "achieved" or "mastered" but can be continuously enhanced and strengthened. They provide an alternate set of lenses on conflict and negotiation that further enriches comprehension and potential outcomes. They are options in the field of choosing and acting. They cannot be measured, artificially created, or contained in category boxes.

Another Disclaimer

I liked the last disclaimer so much I decided to add another. This one is about my own limits. The ways of being I describe here are very difficult for me much of the time. Many times I fail to achieve even a modest manifestation of some of them. I am not writing about them because I am particularly "good" at them, but because when I have been able to express them in my behavior, I have found that the outcomes are creative and constructive. I find that they ask a great deal of me, and sometimes I simply am not equal to the challenge.

I also have been watching my own progression with these ways of being and have noticed that I am at peace personally when I express them. This is attractive to me. I am not always clever enough to seek and achieve my own personal peace, but I am committed to the effort to do so.

I have also noticed how others respond to these ways of being. I would like to assure you that everyone gets wildly thrilled and happy with them and writes me thank-you notes and throws confetti when I walk in the room. This is not the case. Many people join me in my efforts, much good accrues from this, and these people tell me so. This adds great pleasure to my personal peace, and has improved the quality of my life immeasurably. It also brings me great joy to find and experience a community of other persons with whom I can make common cause.

Some people do become very uncomfortable and miss the good old days. This can be a distressing experience but does not appear to be fatal. The struggle to move to new realities is always difficult, and since I regress regularly, I am loathe to deny others the same escape. We are ultimately a fairly vulnerable and frightened lot, we humans.

Some people become very passive when these ways of being are in their vicinity. They sense the call to change, to take responsibility for their own lives, to join in a common effort to create. They are not interested in this call and often have created a reality for themselves where others do for them what they would most constructively do for themselves. They don't really want to give up their dependencies. They may be very quiet, even pleasant in a very hollow kind of manner, but they will not assist you in these ways of being and can often impede the creative process through their passive resistance. They are best left to their own devices, since they can absorb an enormous amount of your time and energy if you try to entice them into a process of no honest interest to them.

A few people become outraged. It is my sense, however, that this last group started out outraged, and I merely served as a catalyst to unearth what was lurking beneath the surface before I ever arrived in their lives. Again, the shadow. I have learned over time that such persons were unlikely to negotiate in good faith. Hence, it sometimes seems like a service to help unveil the outrage. With their masks intact, they wreak havoc on many a sincere group of people.

It has sometimes been very difficult for me to deal with this outrage, and I have not always done so well, but it is a small price to pay compared to the price of manipulative maneuvers. I can say that sort of philosophically, but to tell you the truth, I really hate being attacked and demeaned, so if it seems unattractive to you, I can certainly understand your reaction. It helps to remember and recognize the face of the omnipotent child.

It is probably important to note here that the small proportion of persons who become outraged can also become very destructive and hurtful. While this is not the usual response I experience to these ways of being, it is one of the possibilities. It helps me to remember Ghandi's lesson that only in creating the conditions for potential violence do I master my own impulse to seek revenge, by choosing to not act on this impulse. There are lessons to be learned from the outraged.

I wish I could give you a more enthusiastic and unbridled report on how easy and fun it is to manifest the ten ways of being that you will find discussed here. I don't think all this candor is really bad news, but it is honest news. Having read lots of books that promise me things they truly cannot deliver, I am hopeful that you will at least be encouraged by my realism. I think every human has a light side and a dark side. I think it helps to remember this, especially about myself.

This willingness to mention both the light and dark sides of reality as I experience it is something I struggle with a great deal. Pessimists bore and irritate me, but then so do optimists. I think the pessimists are simply blotting out all the beauty and joy and fun of living, creating realities that structure for the worst possible outcomes. I think optimists deny the difficulty and challenge of human existence, the pain real humans feel and endure. I believe it is possible to work toward transforming all these dark dimensions, but not by escapism, denial, suppression, or aggression. So I trundle along with my struggle for balance, knowing that the pessimists think me too perky and positive and the optimists find me disturbingly willing to note the shadows of the human condition. I suppose my perception of pessimists and optimists as boring and irritating probably doesn't help, but it just shows you how hard it is for me to manifest the ways of being at an uneven table sometimes.

A Further Shift in Reality: The Paradigm Shift

As we edged toward the close of the century, looking back reflectively we noticed that one of the several cataclysmic events we humans shared involved evolutionary shifts that express themselves most dramatically in the theories of relativity. They have had a monumental impact on all of us. We learned that a rich array of factors ultimately determine what you see: where you sit, where you look, how you look, what you look for, at what speed you look, when you look, and why you look. It is hard to get our minds around this idea. We really had hoped we could hold all of this constant, so that all of us would see the same thing. We also often hope that the thing we see is the only thing to be seen, which happily then makes us "right" and everyone else "wrong." It appears it simply isn't that simple. Time magazine named Albert Einstein the "Person of the Century" to remind us of this fact.

Further, one set of givens for looking, if repeated, in some cases, lead to seeing the same thing and in other cases, to seeing something else. This has made us feel a good deal messier than we did a century ago when the hope for unlimited knowledge through science held us in thrall. We also thought we could contain all the information, and have since discovered that unlike coal and crated peaches, information is leaky stuff that spreads about no matter how much we try to contain it. We have even created technology that ensures the leakage.

Then we discovered that "we" were only part of "we" and that there were other communities of humans who saw things quite differently than "we" did in some respects. "We" began to worry, since "we" once thought that "we" all agreed, or would someday agree. "We" took comfort in believing that in time everyone would see things "our" way. Some people said they didn't agree. Some said that they saw completely different things and were quite content to not see what "we" saw. They even claimed "we" might be seeing in a distorted fashion. This was a very troublesome development. We set about to show all the people who didn't see what we saw why they should see what we saw, and how deficient they were if they failed to see what we saw. With our new information technology, we could experience all these conflicts with little or no time lapse, and hence little or no time for reflection.

Thomas Kuhn (1970) wrote a book called *The Structure of Scientific Revolutions* that crystallized some of these issues and proposed an approach to making sense of them. He described the process of changing over that these insights evoke as a "paradigm shift." While many people didn't ever read what Thomas had to say, and many gave some very interesting spins to his ideas, the term itself has become part of our language system in the United States. It is somewhat jargony, and hence I hesitate to use it, but it has utility for me.

For me, a paradigm shift emerges when cultures, groups, or even an individual find themselves unable to explain something with the old answers. The old answers may not apply to something new that has recently been "seen," or to something "seen" for a long time where the old explanation no longer seems adequate. The search for new answers leads to an array of alternatives. Over time, some new explanatory stories begin to enjoy a degree of popularity because they meet the needs of the searchers in one way or another. Sometimes the process occurs in only one or two dimensions of a culture. Other times it may be quite pervasive and touch many dimensions, or disrupt old answers to some of the most compelling and important questions of that culture. At some level, this seems to me another way of describing the evolution we inexorably pursue.

An Exercise

Try this one in your journal. Write down five changes you have experienced in the last five years that you think are pretty substantial ones for you personally. Now write down five global changes that you think are pretty substantial ones for all humans. Assign a number from zero to ten, zero meaning "this disturbs me enormously" and ten meaning "this thrills me enormously" and the other numbers falling somewhere between these extremes.

Now study your numbers. Did anything get a zero or one, or a nine or ten? What does this mean? Did you share this viewpoint with anyone as the change was occurring? If you shared your viewpoint, did you share your emotions also? Did any of your numbers cluster around four, five, or six? Were these really substantive changes for you? If so, why? If not, why not? If you had to write down twenty changes, could you? How much do you change? Do you like to change? What do you do when change is imposed on you by someone else? Do you like to impose change? Do you hate answering these stupid questions about change?

These paradigm shifts don't always make people thrilled with the joy of discovery. If you liked the old answers, no matter how clearly they are now obsolete, it is hard to let go. If you don't like the new answers, your plight is even worse. If you crafted a full and satisfying life around the old answers, the new answers may seem to be hostile forces, dangerous new thoughts. We humans often struggle with change. Since reality is a social construction, the search for a common story or set of answers, or a set of stories that can live comfortably together, is no small challenge. Creating new realities can thus be very risky business.

These ways of being run that risk. I have formally warned you of that fact now, and the choice is yours. I know I don't control your choice, and I also know that you do. I only control the clarity and honesty with which I try to tell you about all of this, and the degree of fidelity I muster in shifting my own way of being into a new paradigm that may enable a more constructive effort toward conflict resolution.

Having said these things, before I describe the ways of being, I want to briefly present my description of the current paradigm shifts I feel that I am experiencing in this culture. They inform my approach to an uneven table, and they are the conceptual backdrop for the ways of being. I have been trying to construct a useful way of describing my sense of these shifts for about twenty years now, and I have even published earlier versions of this description of shifting paradigms. My thinking will no doubt continue to evolve, so I am merely presenting my understanding to this point.

16

A Model of Paradigm Shifts
for the Millennium

My reflections on paradigm shifts for the millennium involve an array of interacting observations and insights. I think that there are many paradigm shifts occurring simultaneously, because part of the old paradigm expressed excessive compartmentalization, where we truly hoped or believed we could put little chunks of reality in boxes or containers and keep them from each other. We somehow hoped physics and anthropology would stay on their own separate turfs, that when we were at work we ceased to have a family for eight hours each day, that our feelings of revulsion at killing people would not bubble up if we didn't have to watch them being killed, that religious tolerance would eventually lead to compassion. What with all these boxes, evolutionary shifts seem to have to go from box to box to break down the artificial separations.

I think that all these paradigm shifts are ultimately the same shift and that they are all connected to one another and potentiating one another. I think that the common substrate that they emerge from is more profound and substantive than the one we have been embracing, and that the shift is welcome for me, albeit difficult and disruptive. I think a rich array of humans with an equally rich array of competencies are trying to understand and communicate these shifts, and they have been my teachers. I acknowledge my debt to each of them.

I think these shifts move us collectively and evolutionarily to a richer, wiser, larger, and deeper vantage point. I do not think they promise or deliver perfection, but only that where we are going is preferable to where we were before or where we are now. I choose to make these shifts, even if I do it very clumsily on occasion. I know I am not alone in this. Others choose to make the shifts and do it clumsily as well. I am grateful to those with whom I can make common cause, and I am comforted that they too struggle and stumble on the path.

I think these shifts aim at balance, at righting an imbalance that does not serve the planet, the people on it, or the dreams we embrace. I think that these paradigm shifts are opening vistas, and that in this new position more is visible and the terrain is more comprehensive. I also think that these shifts introduce us to new meanings of "relating" everything, and this new sense of "relating" is the most difficult aspect of the paradigm shifts. Those with relating skills are advantaged in this changeover; those without them are disadvantaged.

It might be helpful at this juncture to very briefly identify some of the paradigm shifts that I think are happening concurrently. While I would like to credit all the authors who have stimulated my thinking about paradigm shifting, some have had a uniquely powerful impact. None would lay claim to my synthesis of ideas as their own, however. Rather than cite the top fifty thinkers to whom I owe thank-you notes here, I have included some of the books that have proven most catalytic for me in the Recommended Readings at the back of the book. For this second edition, I have added several authors who have further clarified my thinking. So, acknowledging all the help I have received, here is an exemplar list of paradigm shifts that I have compiled from the perspective of a citizen of the United States, from these and other sources:

Emergence of multinationals and a world economy

Systematic exploration of the nature of multiculturalism

Examination of patriarchal structures and their effects

Increased permeability of national boundaries

Identification of ways of knowing other than through science

Resurgence of an interest in spirituality

Emergence of linguistics and cognitive sciences

Changing definitions of civil rights

Networking of the planet with information technologies, particularly with the Internet

Discovery of the limits of traditional science

Chaos and complexity theories

Expansion into outer space

Introduction of Eastern philosophical systems to the Western mind

Changing definitions of health, illness, healing, and curing

Extension of the human life cycle

Expansion of the science of consciousness

Manipulation of genetic materials in diverse life forms

Emergence of creative approaches to understanding creativity

Movement from hierarchical to cooperative organizational structures

Evolution of women's movements, men's movements, and gender study

Explosive political reorganization of Europe, Asia, and Africa

Reconceptualization of time and space

Commitment to world ecosystem protection and maintenance

Creation of the information society

Growth of humanistic and depth psychology

Reemergence of a recognition of mystery and myth

It is perhaps self-evident that all sorts of paradigm shifts are not included here, that some are more public and media-saturated than others, that some attract larger numbers of people's interests than others, and that some are more profound than others. The fact that they all are occurring simultaneously seems foolish to ignore, however, and trying to relate them, one to the other, is no small challenge.

The Evolutionary Process

When I mentally try to describe all of this to myself, I think of it as my personal and social participation in emerging paradigms that I believe call forth a personal and social reconstruction, a reframing of reality. I think that this is an expression of the process of human evolution. That process can be thought of as sequential. This is how I describe that process to myself.

Knowing new things manifests itself in naming the new things. Naming generates new language. Language shared creates new social realities. New social realities are explained and reinforced through the use of metaphors. Metaphors are human constructions. Human constructions persist over time but can and do change. This change reflects human consciousness, curiosity, choice, and context. Thus, evolving, emerging paradigms are by their nature personally transformative and create new knowledge, names, language, social realities, and metaphors.

In my fifty-eight years of living, there are many "new knowledges" that have emerged and dramatically changed my life, only some of which are listed above. To try to list all of these is another book, but I will give you a few examples to demonstrate my point. Before ecology, I threw my tin cans and plastic bottles in the garbage without guilt. Before computer science, a byte was something I did immediately before chewing my food. Before quantum theory, I really thought if I worked hard enough I could know everything and there would be one right answer. Before feminist theory, I thought I was simply confused when some explanations of reality seemed partial or flawed when compared with my experiences. There are others, of course: bioenergetics, megatrends, Russian democracy, collective unconscious, deconstructionism, participative management, genetic reengineering, mythopoetic men's literature, string theory, AIDS immunology, Buddhism, CNN, MTV, and the Bermuda Triangle.

Most of these were simply not part of my educational experience. In day-to-day living, I watched social reality change as these became part of it. New names, new language, and new social realities emerged, essentially without any real effort on my part. They just happened. As a college student, I loved chemistry. I would actually stay up at night to read chemistry books. I thought the periodic chart was a stroke of genius played out before my eyes, and I loved the idea that we had actually figured out the structure of the atom. We humans seemed so clever to me. When I got the news that physicists had discovered quarks, I was crestfallen; I thought I'd been betrayed. Then alpha particles, then beta particles, and today I watch the debate on the supercollider and know that things change in ways we don't fully grasp.

Other new names and languages are our daily bread. Once gender roles were the things we memorized so we could do them right. No one had imagined a hologram, or multiple modes of knowing. Transcendentalism was something occult that we knew separated us from foreign others, and gods and goddesses were not a common topic of concern, but a foray into Greek mythology—the only mythology many of us thought counted. I did not worry about acid rain or black holes or ozone layers, and I did not make phone calls with satellites helping me to do so. The behavior of oppressed groups and the shadow functions of the personality did not worry me as a child, despite active involvement in both. AIDS were things people did when they helped others out. As a culture, we chose not to even notice our racism, and wanted to believe that somehow Martin Luther King Jr. had solved the whole issue in a tidy fashion. We seemed to have no idea that it could actually become more complex than before.

Writing about these things makes me feel like a relic. Most of the names and knowledges I am describing are quite recent, however, and all of them have embedded in them very substantive social changes. In a culture that has been and sometimes still wishes to be habituated to the "one right way," these new names signal new forms of discomfort, new social realities that will inevitably disrupt the old ones. Most of these new things just refuse to cram themselves into our old models of reality.

From Either/Or to Both/And

Had we been a social system that enjoyed diversity, that reveled in the mix, that made the melting pot more than merely a sentimental metaphor, we might not have felt so nervous about all these things. But in the main, we are a culture that likes a right answer, and when a second answer emerges, we seek to find an answer between what we consider competing alternatives. If we cannot see one prevailing truth, we set up a countertruth force and create a competition. At some level, we indeed create a conflict.

The seduction of dualistic thinking is powerful for all of us. If you add to that a deeply felt interest in establishing dominance and control, it is not difficult to understand what our most spontaneous response to two seemingly mutually exclusive ideas will be. It is no accident that we seem stuck in the image of a "two-party system." We like conflict. Sometimes we even call it free enterprise. And like kids on a corner lot, we like one-on-one, and may the best "man" win. For us, life is an either/or proposition, not a both/and adventure. As physicians have been telling me for years, "What you nurses need to understand is that someone has to be in charge of everything." It has never escaped my attention that the someone apparently wasn't me.

Given our fascination with competition and conflict, dominance and control over everything, all these new realities we created had to either cleverly slide themselves into the existing structures, or stand outside of them. If one could not slide them in, if they stood outside, they would then run the risk of being experienced as challenges to the existing structures. Indeed, in some cases, they sought to do exactly that. To the extent that they succeeded, they did not necessarily become cherished, but often more shrilly troublesome. Watching the varied responses to the competence and character of Anita Hill and Hillary Rodham Clinton has been instructive in this regard.

These existing structures have certain characteristics. These always seem obvious to me, but they still sometimes make people uncomfortable when I say them out loud, as if naming them unveils their true nature. Nonetheless, they need to be described at this point. They are primarily patriarchal in nature, assuming that the best model of leadership available requires a man who optimally functions as a kindly but firm father who will control others. They are hierarchical, assuming various prescribed levels of power and control over others. They focus on dominant power and control as a central source of meaning, as a goal worthy to be sought, and once attained, retained.

They are largely materialistic and tend to deny, ignore, or discount dimensions of reality that cannot be visibly seen, measured, or controlled. They emphasize mechanistic processes, using a rational and analytical mode of discourse. They change and prosper through a process of argumentation. Competing and prevailing, carried to the extreme of war, they provide the preferred model of change and are the stuff of human history. They are largely predicated on the value of being nationalistic. The dilemma of creating world peace by serving as an international police force is a useful exemplar of this viewpoint, as are our domestic "wars" on drugs, poverty, AIDS, and violence.

These structures unveil our country's dominant paradigm, one that is largely analytical, linear, causal, reductionistic, hierarchical, and focused on observables. This is a "way of being." We are interested in controlling things—actually, just about everything. We therefore seek predictive knowledge and aim to make it objectified and quantifiable. And we want to win at any cost.

We prefer scientific knowledge to just about any other kind of knowing, and actively discredit or trivialize all other ways of knowing We ask science to solve all of our problems, and we use the central tool of competition among theories to identify the answer we select. We believe this is the best way, even when the results are troublesome or inadequate. We need science to win. Science, we believe, gives us control of everything. It declares us the force in control of the knowing and defines the known as a powerless "it". We do not think that this way of knowing is ever in question, only that our methods are not yet refined enough. We trust science in the same way that people trusted religion in the Middle Ages, and we believe that it should and will prevail. We believe that we have found nothing better.

By now, you may be wondering where this is all leading. It gets a bit heavyhanded, I know, so I think it might be fun to take a time-out and do an exercise. This will give you a chance to get to know this dominant paradigm in a nice personal way.

An Exercise

Take a few moments and reflect on some of the social structures that you spend time in day to day. It might be your family, or your extended family, or your job, or a club or organization you belong to. It might be your neighborhood or your school or your church. Picture yourself there. You might want to write down the answers to the questions I'm going to raise, just for the fun of it.

Who's in charge? Does whoever is in charge have some people who report to him or her? And do others report to those persons? Do any of these people exercise power over you? Do they control you? If you are one of the persons in charge, do you control others? What do you do with your time there—what do you talk about, deal with, spend time on? How do you go about doing this? What do you do when there is a disagreement or a conflict? How is it resolved? Do you think that everyone else in the United Sates does things this same way? Do you think people in Indonesia, Kenya, or Peru do things this same way? Do you know the answer to the last question? Do you want to know the answer to the last question?

If someone suggested that the first thing we all need to do to figure out the answers to these questions was to see how we "feel" about them, what our deepest emotions are about them, and to talk about that openly and in some depth, what would you think of this proposal? Would it be attractive to you, comfortable, meaningful? Would you welcome the opportunity? How would you know if you got closer to some answer to all of these questions? Do you hope I quit asking these questions pretty soon?

If a new paradigm is emerging, how does it differ from this "life-as-usual" image, this dominant paradigm? This may or may not require a stretch of your imagination, depending on how much time you spend thinking about the changes going on around you. Some people ponder these things out of curiosity. Others believe that they are forced to do so because of life changes. Some brave and clever people simply choose to live a full and vibrant life, and that means staying open to all the possibilities.

What if, in addition to analyzing a problem, taking it apart, and looking at all the pieces, we were equally captivated by the variety of ways we could find relationships between all the pieces, equally curious about diverse ways of bringing the pieces together in creative new relationships, of synthesizing new wholes from various parts? What if, in addition to seeing the linear process, we were fascinated as much by the networks of relationships among linear processes, found the matrix as interesting as the equation, and in doing so discovered that there were forces still not admitted into the matrix? What if we not only wanted to isolate a problem so we could solve it, but found it equally fascinating to look at the problem in context, in all the ways it is embedded in a variety of realities, related to absolutely everything else? What if we were willing to consciously experience that, knowing full well that many dimensions of reality were beyond our comprehension?

The richest exploration of this emerging paradigm that I have found is the work being done by the Institute of Noetic Sciences (IONS). Astronaut Edgar Mitchell, its founder, describes the sciences emerging from this paradigm. These sciences explore a universe that is learning, self-organizing, adaptive, creative, trial and error, intelligent, aware, evolving, unpredictable, and expanding (Mitchell, 1998). His description stands in stark contrast to the dominant paradigm.

An example may be useful here. Willis Harman, a former president of the IONS board of directors, addressed the limits of the dominant paradigm in a series of monographs, one focused on re-examining the metaphysical foundations of modern science (Harman, 1991). He notes that among other anomalies that modern science fails to address adequately, there is no place for the consciousness of the observer, expressed, for instance, in the volition of the observer. This warrants reflection. How can the scientist, while exercising consciousness, pretend it does not exist, has no impact? The interest in control and prediction emerges from a specific type of consciousness. The dominant paradigm thus sustains a reality map unequal to its own challenge, one that fails to acknowledge its own inherent practices.

We might begin to acknowledge that we don't control everything. We might even discover that control constricts, and that the creative moment moves beyond predicted possibilities. We might want to create some models of managing things where relationship was as significant a force as hierarchical structures. Rather than seeking to control, we might seek to relate, and focus on the patterns and processes that might enable that. We might even begin to imagine multiple ways of knowing, and discover new dimensions of the power of ethical knowing or aesthetic knowing or intuitive knowing. These are traits of emerging paradigms.

I hope you noticed, however, that I didn't want to throw out the old paradigm. It has some utility. It gave you and me penicillin and rayon; it can't be all bad. But I want more. I want it when it fits, and other options when it doesn't fit. It seems a burdened old paradigm, carrying all of reality around on its shoulders, and it is clearly unequal to the task. It's desperate need to "be right about everything" is systematically suppressing its innovative potential. It seems strapped in its own rigidity and refusal to see what it cannot control. I think emerging paradigms give us the option of expansion, creativity, freedom, largeness of scope. If we must insist on dualism, they give us balance.

Conceptualized in this fashion, the emerging paradigm gives us access to some forces that would address the imbalance of a dominant paradigm and lead to a social reconstruction of reality. This could benefit us all. We would not need to confine ourselves to patriarchal structures but could have structures led by the person most fit to do the job, for that hour or week or month or year. Sometimes we would implement hierarchies, and sometimes we would implement more fluid and interactive matrix organizations, where predictions of outcomes were sometimes considered deterrents to creative new relationships. We could imagine that human worth or potential could evoke at least as much persuasive interest as power and control. Our mechanistic bent could be tempered by a more holistic worldview; our materialistic bent tempered by a more humanistic worldview. We might imagine ourselves collaborating where once only argumentation and competition prevailed. In a moment of rashness, we might even begin to think global thoughts.

Crafting New Metaphors

To achieve this, we would have to begin to honestly assess our current metaphors and observe how many reduce to images designed to sustain and reinforce the dominant paradigm. While we may continue to use the metaphors of war, argumentation, domination, and control, we might also imagine metaphors about creating, cooperating, relating, and connecting. Some that have sometimes proven helpful to me include weaving, making a tapestry, conducting an orchestra, quilting, healing, ocean waves, growing, gardening, and journeying. I personally have a fondness for one that permits me to "keep the dance going!" As T. S. Eliot observes, "there is only the dance" (1943, p. 16).

Now that I've deluged you with dualistic images, I need to acknowledge that I really think it's a great deal more multiple and complex than this, but if we want to search for balance, we need to imagine and begin. When I tried to imagine and begin, I went in search of an analogue. We use metaphors to learn. I finally settled on the image of a DNA molecule. It is pictured in the center of Figure 16.1 as an image revealing a set of relationships. If all the dominant paradigm forces were to be altered not by destruction but by complementarity, one could envision a creative alternative to conflict that sought to create DNA molecules of relationship and balance. I like it. Actually, I like it enough that you're not obliged to do so. It might however start a conversation in your head. In Figure 16.1, I have tried

Figure 16.1. Paradigm Dimensions by "DNA Strand."

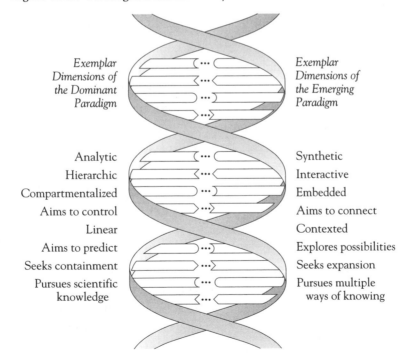

Exemplar Dimensions of the Dominant Paradigm	Exemplar Dimensions of the Emerging Paradigm
Analytic	Synthetic
Hierarchic	Interactive
Compartmentalized	Embedded
Aims to control	Aims to connect
Linear	Contexted
Aims to predict	Explores possibilities
Seeks containment	Seeks expansion
Pursues scientific knowledge	Pursues multiple ways of knowing

to indicate what might be found on each of the two strands of the DNA, the double helix of Watson fame. I think this is my metaphorical nod to the genome project.

I have already shared parts of this with several different audiences and individuals over the years, and one of the ways it creates discomfort is that we become confused about the idea of complementarity. Some view it as dependency. They assume that they can only embrace one "half" of the DNA molecule, and hence they must ask others to embrace the other side on their behalf, to do for them what they can, perhaps must do for themselves if they actually wish for fullness and wholeness of being. Some think that the "good" trait we wish to sustain will have to be destroyed to manifest its obverse. We fear that if the "other side" of the double helix is equally credible, is to be given serious consideration and air time, that this will diminish the side we hang out on. We fear diminishment through competition rather than recognizing enrichment through abundance. We subtly embrace a zero-sum game, even if the physicists tell us that the universe is constantly expanding. We use some pretty emotionally unattractive words to sustain this confusion.

Some examples might help here. We think the obverse of giving is withholding, when it is more promising to imagine it as receiving. We think the obverse of discriminating is being indiscriminate, when it is more creative to imagine it as being inclusive. We think that the obverse of active is passive, when it might also be thought of as receptive. We think that the obverse of rational is irrational, when it might better be viewed as intuitive. We think of the obverse of initiating as the lack of initiative, when it might also be thought of as responsiveness. We think of the obverse of disciplined as undisciplined, while it might also be self-accepting. We think of the obverse of gentleness as harshness, but it might also be imagined as forcefulness. Opposites confound, create forced choices, evoke conflict. Obverses refer to the sides of a coin, to the "counterpart necessarily involved in or answered to a fact or truth," as the dictionary puts it. In Figure 16.2, I have tried to provide the image

Figure 16.2. Complementarity: An Alternate Viewpoint on a Range of Contrasts Between Human Traits.

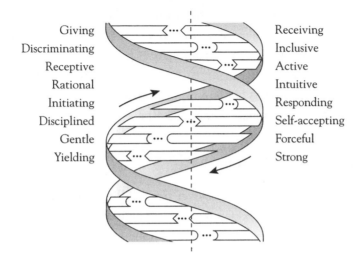

Giving	Receiving
Discriminating	Inclusive
Receptive	Active
Rational	Intuitive
Initiating	Responding
Disciplined	Self-accepting
Gentle	Forceful
Yielding	Strong

of such obverses as they might relate to a DNA relational image, where two manifestations interact and interweave.

Which is to say, if we want to create a paradigm that both honors the strength and contributions of our dominant paradigm, yet creates changes that portend something more robust and promising for us all, we can achieve this by balancing the dimensions of the dominant paradigm with their obverses—the dimensions that are overshadowed. The biggest challenge with a dominant paradigm in our culture is that we are so either/or that letting it get tempered with the "balancing obverse" is hard to imagine. Better we just bomb the thing, we mutter to ourselves. Or, if we love it dearly, we must protect it to the death. The war imagery is deliberate here. It captures my sense of how we respond. It is not an accident that when we try to identify the opposites of the things we cling to and cherish, we often use words with hostile or negative connotations. "Uppity" black people and "ball breaking" women know that those who use these designations would value them more if they were passive and compliant, and may do them harm if they refuse. A dominant paradigm that has imbedded in its assumptions a belief in "one right way" is inherently vulnerable and defensive, particularly if it must deny substantial dimensions of reality to sustain the belief.

Over time, I have learned that this is indeed the most troublesome aspect of our dominant paradigm. It posits the need to prevail, and hence renders us reluctant or seemingly unable to balance obverses in the interest of harmony or even simple intellectual clarity. It seems to me a uniquely vulnerable aspect of Western traditions.

Embracing the Paradox

Being unbalanced is neither clever nor fulfilling. This is not a stunning insight. Yet introducing anything new in our country, where we switch to power and dominance concerns without even consciously recognizing it, is fraught with difficulty. Finding some new imagery for creating new social realities that do not completely destroy the old would be an interesting adventure. If we watch the decline of the Eastern European bloc and the travails of this process, we might learn something of merit. This does not look like an attractive model for change to me.

I think of many of the dimensions of the emerging paradigm as the "silent dimensions" of what it means to be human. They are silent because we thought we could only have one dimension, and we have been systematically cheating ourselves out of these other dimensions, silencing them in ourselves and in others. Many were relegated to or captured by those who have not been parties to the dominant paradigm. Hence, often, some people at uneven tables have significant ability in some aspects of these silent dimensions and can offer them as a resource in seeking a balanced resolution to our conflicts. If we were to create DNA relational models, both forces would be valued. If we were to create DNA relational models, the balance would be the goal, not prevailing or victory. However, to do so we would have to find a way to evoke, to give voice to the silent dimension. And we would have to choose to listen.

We would also have to know that the goal of giving voice to the silent dimensions is not to harm others less able or to prevail over them, but to create balance. The emerging paradigm could conceivably move toward complementarity rather than dominance, could fill out the tapestry rather than replacing it, could swell the music of the symphony rather than silencing Mozart as an act of deference to Bach or silencing the violins as an act of deference to the oboes. We could choose balance over competition, and would then make manifest the greatest strength of that which is coming forth. To pass legislation that protects women without noting that it harms men, or further justice for ethnic minorities while perpetrating injustice on those who are not is simply recycling the dominant paradigm with new players. It is not social change at its best.

Evolution does not seem to be something any one person or group of people control. We are stumbling toward some new expressions through the emerging paradigm, no matter how much the advocates of the dominant paradigm resist these changes or how confused the voices of the silent dimensions become. I did not expect that I would live to see the Berlin Wall come down, no matter how much I had hoped for this. I do not think I can find the meaning of dying from AIDS, no matter how much I wish I could give this gift to others. There is still mystery, and I find myself more whole for honoring that fact. More simplistically, we can either figure out how to live together and value and celebrate the variance, enriching ourselves with it, or we can blow up the planet. The choice always seems sort of straightforward to me.

As someone trained from birth in the abilities and insights of the silent dimension, I have been struck by how intensely many people work to keep them silent. I have been startled at the efforts some people will go through to keep the silent silenced. Sometimes it seems so desperate it seems funny, other times it seems sad, and occasionally it seems frankly destructive and self-destructive. By the time I figured much of this out for myself, I had aged considerably. It took me a while to retrieve the lost dimensions.

the reclamation project

using intermittent tracings of
captive remembrance,
i'm out in search of
fragments of myself
that passed no one's inspection,

shards of orchid jardinieres,
clay pot clutter,
shelved in the pawn shops
of my loves and lovers.

i'm moving like some homeless hag
craving bag lady status,
a crone fingering remnants, selecting
from a cache of silent, solemn
memories

crushed and mingled on racks
in unlit resale shops
run by brittle blue-haired ladies
who wear scarlet nails and pendletons.

i'm sifting through the garbage sites
of human refuse
(souls, tears, terror and stuff)
looking for odd coinage,
archaic currencies,

slices and slivers of forgotten and
momentary offerings, scattered
like ashes on beach and sea,
leveled in shapeless landfills.

i'm washing ashore like driftwood, mixed
with scraps of stormy lake histories,
senseless, nameless dumpings
of muddy seaweed, stalks, stones,
and urban litter,

here barely used,
here somewhat overused,
somewhat beyond repair:
immobilized.

i will not soon once more
catch the wind and
toss my soul
with such complete
release and sweet abandon.

no more promises to make or keep.
    —pbk

Giving Voice to an Alternative Reality

I have taken the time to draw this admittedly condensed, yet perhaps over long picture of the alternate reality that guides me for a very specific reason. Using my metaphors, it is the score from which the orchestra performs for me, or the loom on which I do my weaving. It is an essential facet of the process for me. If one would take the ways of being described here, and attempt to make them the tools of sustaining the dominant paradigm or ensuring that the emerging paradigm defeated the dominant paradigm, they simply would be of no utility. In fact, I think they would prove to be quite destructive. I am trying to say this as plainly as I can, since I think it is important. I did not go to the trouble of writing this book to introduce power purveyors to ten more ways of manipulating reality for purposes of control and dominance. As you can see, this worries me.

I also sense that while many people with whom I've shared these images find them valuable, they also find them difficult. I do too. Yet if we want to address conflict despite the persistence of an uneven table and our virtual fixation on dominance power, to have some difficult ways of being may be better than none—or better than the traditional ones. They have proven their utility to me, and I am eager to have conversations with others about them.

It will no doubt amaze you to discover that I am finally going to tell you about the ten ways of being at an uneven table. But first this!

A Story

My daughter Becky, in her third year of life and second year in a university day-care center, became known as the child who could best help integrate new students who could not speak English. I was vaguely aware of this and had a lot of respect for Becky's gregariousness, but I thought little else about it. One day, as we arrived, the head teacher in her room very matter-of-factly asked me to take Becky to the main office as soon as she put her things away. They were waiting for her because they had a new student who could not speak any English. Becky was equally unimpressed with the request and headed for the front office. This caught my attention. It seemed pretty unusual to me, and I began to reflect on this unusualness.

I thought about it all day, off and on, and wondered what exactly she did. Musing, I thought she probably taught them how to say yes and no first, then maybe table or chair or bathroom or food or water. Perhaps she taught them toy, door, outside, playground. By the time I picked her up that evening, I had a fairly elaborate collection of assumptions. Knowing my role, however, I came as student and asked her how she did it.

"Well, first I teach them how to say Becky, and I make them practice over and over again until they get it right." I was shocked! Wow, was my kid self-centered! Here was this poor stranger in a strange land, and my kid was imprinting her own dear name as the first, central, and most powerful word for mastery of the foreign tongue. I managed not to give my spontaneous speech on humility, as if I knew something of it, and asked her why she did that.

"Well, these kids are really scared, Mom, and really alone, and they can't talk to anyone or anything. It's awful, and mostly no one really understands them. The first thing they need to know is that they have a friend, you know, a kid like me, and so they need to know my name. That way, if anything awful happens or they get real scared or upset, they just have to say my name and then the teacher comes and gets me and I stay with them and try to help them so they're not so scared and alone. That way everyone knows that they should just come and get me. Sometimes they get really upset and cry and everything or they throw fits, so I just try to figure out what's wrong when I get there, and sometimes I just hug them."

———————

17

Way of Being Number One

Find and Inhabit the Deepest and Surest Human Space That Your Capabilities Permit

While dominance power and control over others is given substantive value in our culture, many other dimensions of what it means to be human are equally or more compelling for most people. Examples of this might include loving one's children and leaving them a decent legacy, or respecting one's own intrinsic worth as a human, or protecting a fragile environment. These deeper and surer things are not necessarily about life's ultimates, but may include simple things like a pleasant workplace or a clean neighborhood. When you start thinking about deeper and surer things, you might be surprised at how many things actually do mean a great deal more to you than controlling someone or something.

Compared to the simple exercise of dominant power, these deeper and surer dimensions of what it means to be a human may often ask more of us, but also give us a great deal more. They can improve the quality of our lives and the lives of others. And, happily enough, they can provide supplemental or even alternative emphases in negotiations. For persons who elect to sit at an uneven table, they provide a vantage point that eliminates reducing oneself to bickering over dominant power. Since the uneven table may be set with the assumption that we cannot exercise dominant power anyway, this gives us a reason to be at the table that goes beyond watching someone habituated to dominant power sustain his or her habit.

Trusting the Human Spirit

In attempting to explore this way of being, I have found that it is sometimes difficult for me to introduce these issues when I know I am at a table where they might be viewed as naïve or sentimental, rather than as compelling or substantive. Because I am a woman, others' responses to them are sometimes "reduced" to a patronizing nod to "women's issues," which tend to then be defined as lovely but irrelevant. I have been startled to find how introducing the ethical dimension of a conflict, for instance, can sometimes be considered in bad taste, as if I had failed to outgrow some developmental stage where profound things moved me.

Yet I have also experienced a great hunger in many people for a more compelling vision of reality. We have neglected, dismantled, and abused the dimensions of humanness that most enrich the human spirit, or have turned them into peripheral or lifeless forms. For many people, I find that reintroducing access to these visions can be a welcome opportunity. Many people would like to take a time-out from cynicism and express what really counts for them. They are often too frightened or too proud to do so, but we have not yet totally silenced this interest in our own inherent capacity for depth of character. I have found that inviting people to a more robust agenda provides options and may evoke or catalyze their imagination, too. Bringing to a negotiation a focus on what is best about the human spirit often activates that best dimension in others.

A Story

For several years, I taught nursing in a variety of state psychiatric institutions. Often these hospitals were merely "holding tanks" where persons abandoned by society and their own families were provided with little that gave life meaning. One such hospital had a ward where persons arrested for a variety of offenses were subsequently hospitalized, either to be evaluated for a psychiatric illness or because they were medically diagnosed as having one.

It was standard procedure to admit these persons, mostly men, by bringing them into a large central room on the unit where most of the patients spent their leisure time and then removing their handcuffs in a somewhat ceremonial fashion. This practice was not only demeaning to the patient, but a painful reminder of past experiences for all of the patients. My students and I decided that there might be an option or an alternative.

We began exploring this with the various decision makers. The more we explored, the more it became clear that the reason for this ceremony was often punitive humiliation and control of the other patients by reminding them of their plight. The assumption was that this served both as a deterrent to the other persons and also reminded the new resident of "his origins." It was ultimately a hostile gesture.

We elected to discuss it in the group meetings held each day with the patients. As we shared our view that the new patient might be benefited to find this a place where helpfulness was as pervasive as punitiveness, the other patients began to speak forcefully about their agreement with this, and their desire to create that message. They noted that they would try to be helpful to this patient if the practice were discontinued.

At first with reluctance, the staff agreed. The patients were so pleased with the call to be more human to one another that they worked very hard to keep their word. Soon the new practice of admitting patients privately, in a separate office, became common, and people quickly forgot both the old practice and its rationale.

While the negotiations for this took some time, the eventual humanizing of the unit was well worth the struggle. In addition, the patients, who had an excellent communication network, were grateful to me and my students and showed that gratitude in a variety of constructive ways. It became amusing to me that after receiving the daily professional report when I came on the unit, I would then be taken aside by one of the patients to be given the "real report" about what was going on, who was upset, why he was upset, and what we might want to do about it. I quickly learned that this report better reflected the needs and hopes of the patients.

During my years as a psychiatric nurse educator, I have had repeated experiences of this kind with people who were supposedly disturbed and dangerous. It has given me a very deep respect for the hunger of the human spirit for something beyond compulsions about control. My awareness of this way of being as constructive actually emerged from my own fatigue and boredom at being at tables where the repetitive struggle for power dominated the entire process. It has always struck me as a fairly lifeless process, predictable and without any significant creative potential.

Over time, I learned to start avoiding such tables, even if I did not experience myself as disadvantaged. I started only wanting to go to tables where I had some assurance that I could experience something more than the tediousness of power negotiations. I started picking my tables, and the ones I selected were ones where the common goal—or the one I introduced—was about issues that were more interesting, more creative, and more engaging. Invariably, they created new realities that made a good deal more sense than what had preceeded them, and they were always more rewarding. If I am at a table where I know I am defined as more powerless than others, it takes a bit more courage to raise these issues, but I have learned over time to trust the capacity for depth in others and the importance of substantive issues to them.

A Story

One of the ways that nursing instructors attempt to create collaborative relationships with the health care environments where they teach is to give something back to those environments. Since both practicing nurses and nursing faculty are so blatantly exploited in so many situations, this mutuality has a creativity about it that often exceeds one's hopes.

Early in my teaching career, I agreed to give a presentation to a state hospital nursing staff. I was naïve about such agreements, though, and squirmed when I discovered that I was to give a talk on "violence and physical danger" with psychiatric patients. It was to be a mandatory presentation for all staff, which meant they would be there because they were forced to be there.

I knew this hospital well enough to know that many of their mandatory educational programs were boring, preachy, and showed little sensitivity to the challenges actually faced by the staff. They were often designed to make the educator feel superior or more intelligent or to convince everyone that the short staffing, poor resources, and inadequate services for these most indigent of clients were acceptable practices. I knew most staff didn't like this, and I shared that viewpoint. I had been a staff nurse in exactly the situation they faced.

Academic communities in this country often lose their sense of mission somewhere along the road and give greater credence to the appearance of cleverness or intelligence than to the substantive ability to assist others in discovering their own passion for the truth. I suddenly faced exactly that dilemma. I was and have always been appalled at the fact that psychiatric nurses literally risk their lives with agitated patients and no one seems to even acknowledge this, let alone help them deal with the situation. Many nurses are assaulted and injured, some for life. It is treated as unfortunate but to be expected. The nonchalance about this offends me deeply.

There have been many interesting studies about this situation. There is a great deal written about an ideal way of addressing this situation. No one, however, writes about how it feels to be the only nurse on a unit with ten, fifteen, or even thirty people at midnight, knowing that several of the patients are violent. I have been there. Writers like to theorize about how this might best be handled. When you read what they write, you know they've never been there.

Here I was, a new faculty member, eager to be viewed as academically competent by the hospital community and my university colleagues. I could viscerally feel the temptation to recite what was in the books, even though I knew it would be of little or no use to anyone. It would only make me look like I had studied all the books. Still, I was seduced. Then I realized how I would fail all those courageous nurses who were facing real violence. So I got up and said what I thought might actually help, what had helped me, what I thought helped most agitated patients. Most of it was not in the books but was about how people might solve problems confronted by violent patients and vulnerable nurses.

I have to admit I was neither cocky nor confident. I felt like I was donating my scholarly credibility to the nearest garbage can. I was anxious and uncertain, but proceeded. At the end, a nurse's aide about twice my width and age came up to me, hugged me spontaneously, and said, "I've been working here and been forced to come to these things for twenty years, honey, and that's the first time someone said something worthwhile that I could really use on the unit!" That hug changed my career.

Taking Risks

There are, however, real risks in this way of being. Many people experience the introduction of more substantive issues as dissonant and may need to practice learning to think about and talk about important things. If they came to the table prepared to negotiate about who gets to control everything and suddenly find themselves discussing the principles on which we will make decisions that will benefit the next generation, they can feel ill-equipped and disoriented. They may have only rarely considered the needs of the next generation as a motive and may want to eliminate such concerns as not germane.

Some people try to "fake" being committed to larger issues. They talk a good show, but only for appearance's sake, to make an impression. Often this is theoretical veiling, and they are eager to seem committed or caring, but equally eager to avoid experiential knowledge. Sometimes people like to talk about issues precisely so no action need be taken. One can usually identify these persons, since they rarely follow through with concrete demonstrations of their comments. Then this merely becomes another variant on manipulation.

There is a problem embedded here. Our culture confuses facticity with wisdom. We emphasize the accumulation of knowledge but fail to develop the gift of wisdom. People with knowledge make great partners for Trivial Pursuit, but they are rarely of value in addressing profound human dilemmas. This is perhaps why struggling for deeper is difficult, since it requires the reflection time that brings forth wisdom. We may have failed to structure our lives so that reflection is as predictable a part of it as brushing our teeth. Once we do, however, we begin to be useful participants in the effort to find deeper and surer ways of attending to conflict.

Committing to Personal Authenticity

This is also the only way to attend to personal authenticity, which is imperative in this way of being. There is a risk here, too, because you have to be willing to own your own "garbage." If people are struggling to move to deeper and surer places, or if they simply don't want to go there, they will ask you to prove or demonstrate your personal authenticity repeatedly. This often feels like shadow projection to me, as if they were saying, "I don't feel authentic enough to deal with this, and I don't want to own my own garbage, so that must be true of you, too. I will prove I am right by putting all of your garbage on the table and trying to prove that you will fail to own it." Developing your own intuitive powers so that you can discriminate about this response in others can be helpful. You also have to be ready when all your garbage sits strewn on the table with everyone staring at it.

All this calls for a type of courage that embraces the best in the meaning of human despite the dangers and deterrents. I myself find I have to fight for this courage nearly every time. It is difficult to come to a table where many people define you as inferior, stupid, defective, or powerless and stay courageously grounded in your own sense of your authentic worth. It becomes harder when they bring your vulnerabilities to the table to discredit your efforts. It takes staying power.

One of the nice things about being perceived as powerless at an uneven table, however, is that you have so little to lose. No one

views you as having power, deserving power, or being a serious con-
tender for power. As a nurse and a woman, I am always amazed at
how blatantly people assume I'm incapable of observing the power
machinations, the patronizing tones, the injustices, and the assumptions about my intellectual incapacities. What I have learned, however, is that this gives me a great deal of freedom to move the
discussion to a deeper and surer place, since I usually have no dominance power or status to claim, protect, or regain. I think this is
one of the really underrated dimensions of being at an uneven table.
Sometimes it is even funny.

A Story

I once attended a conference on improving access to health care in the
United States. It was sponsored by two medical schools, and nearly all of
those in attendance were physicians. I was the only nurse. I sat near the back
and tried to grasp the particular frame that was given to this discussion,
which alternately focused on the inadequacy of salaries for physicians who
gave care to underserved groups, the policies needed to get more medical
students interested in these lower salaries, and the national changes likely to
create different models of care and better salaries through funding subsidies
for graduate medical education.

It sobered me a great deal, and I mused on how my colleagues in nursing were more likely to talk about how to set up a nurse-managed clinic with
little or no funds, which I was then in the process of doing, or changing legislation so certified nurse midwives could prescribe medications independently, which I was then in the process of supporting legislatively. It all
seemed quite strange to me, and I wondered how these physicians would
react to our discussions. I wondered if any of them would ever openly sit
through one, or if they imagined how I was reacting.

Toward the end of the first day, I was asked about my reactions and
shared some of my observations with a small group of the participants, who
were both receptive and open. The next day, the last speaker, a man I knew
personally, began to describe some theoretical approaches to restructuring

the ways we delivered care. Quite spontaneously, and obviously forgetting that I was there, he ended his proposal with "and then we could get the nurses to do the scut work and see how it would work." Half the room spontaneously turned around and stared at me to see what I would do. Two of the physicians asked me to comment.

I attempted, as best I could, to address the comment, uncomfortable and startled by its overtness. What occurred to me retrospectively was how effectively this speaker had raised the awareness of the group in a totally unintentional fashion. There was something funny about this event, and I could laugh at it with others, despite the message it conveyed.

This story actually has an instructive sequel. Several months later, the conference proceedings were sent to me for editing and approval. His comment had been edited out; my response was completely missing and a note advised me it had not been captured by the tape recorder. The speaker, whom I met often after that, was never again fully comfortable in my presence and was often hostile if I raised issues that I believe reminded him of this careless slip. He had apologized at the time of the conference, but I believe he was more disturbed by his public error than the evidence it gave that he needed to reflect on his values. He subsequently became actively involved as a consultant in crafting the new initiatives in health care reform at the national level. I often reflect on this.

———————

Those for whom the focus on dominance power is of great importance often find the introduction of any other focus very disturbing, especially if they simply like the contest or they were certain of winning. Then the desire to keep the negotiation focused on dominance power becomes very intense and does not yield readily to change. If these persons feel threatened by the introduction of additional dimensions, they may attack you. This is not nice but it does happen, and I think it is best to say so. You need to be prepared for this, or you may find yourself counterattacking. Dominance power can be very seductive, especially when you know you could outspar the person attacking you. I experience this as a persistent challenge, since I have found myself sitting with persons so often who assume, based on stereotypical assumptions about women and nurses, that I am far dumber than I actually am. To choose to stay with deeper and surer asks a lot sometimes.

A common form of attack is to try to cheapen or trivialize that which is neither cheap nor trivial, to reduce issues such as justice, truthfulness, compassion, sensitivity, and honesty to niceties that simply have no place in this blood-and-guts, hardball world. After all, it's a jungle out there and we have to operate accordingly. I'm always a bit amazed that no one notices that we are keeping the jungle operative by living by the laws of the jungle, that we create our own reality and actively sustain it when we forgo the opportunity to move to some deeper and surer place.

I have also been told that trying to introduce that which could take us to a surer or deeper place is unrealistic and impossible, that it is nice in theory but simply not feasible. Usually a list of deterrents is then offered as if they were mountains to move rather than realities to change. If you listen closely, there is often a good deal of dominance power lurking in the foothills of those mountains.

Years of attempting to introduce surer or deeper places has taught me that on occasion resistance to moving can become an obsession for others, leading to a virulent campaign of opposition and conflict. While this only happens rarely, it warrants mention, since this type of fixation can become extremely harmful to everyone at the table. This may occur, however, and may indicate that this is a table to leave.

Increasing Self-Awareness

As may be apparent, this particular way of being calls on you to seek more and more self-awareness. You need to be comfortable with self-honesty and self-confrontation. If not, the areas of vulnerability that you deny or ignore become places where your fears can be activated, hence the pathway to discount you so that your ideas can be discounted. Since this is a way of being, it is, I believe, a somewhat endless process. I have found, however, that personal fulfillment makes the process well worth the trouble, and each struggle for greater self-awareness increases my sense of personal security and freedom. I am not more perfect, but I am less amazed at my flaws and less afraid of others noting them. This too can be disturbing to people, however, since they hope that you collapse when confronted with criticism. Agreement with the criticism is frustrating to them and can increase their attacks. This needs to be acknowledged.

Lessons of humility are also embedded in this way of being. Because trying to introduce surer and deeper issues often evokes discrediting behavior, you can quickly discover how well you deal with injured pride and vanity. I personally have found over the years that often I don't deal with these injuries all that well, and when I deteriorate into a frenzy of self-defensiveness or counterattacking, I tend to abandon and others further ignore the surer and deeper issues. This is worth reflecting on a bit. If I can't really be where this way of being asks me to be in a given situation, I may have to simply face that fact. This is a nice solid confrontation with the limits of human nature. In time it can increase your sense of realism. It's just hard to face some days. It is far wiser to face it, and your limits, however, than to indulge in self-deceptions that wreak further havoc. Some days you just need to stay away from uneven tables, and some tables will never be safe for you until you are more secure.

Another subtle insight about surer and deeper merits a bit of reflection. One often reads about conflict resolution as focused on the interests of the parties, with limited attention given to the scope and depth of the interests and the fact that some interests are more profound and compelling than others. Usually there is an assumption that the interests will be pretty self-centered and narcissistic, and little can be done about this. One of the more profound insights of emerging paradigms is that my self-interest is ultimately connected to everyone else's, that if I neglect the interest of others it will eventually have an impact on my well-being. Ecology demonstrates this well. So does poverty manifested as haphazard frustration, rage, and violence. The fabric of society, of the global community, is one piece. To harm one dimension will in time harm us all. We are not used to framing our interests in these lights. We need to try to do so, however, if we hope to grapple with the challenge of surer and deeper negotiations.

Being in Your Place

I have tried to provide a fairly detailed description of this way of being for a reason. I have found that it needs to be a point of departure at an uneven table. The other ways of being become distorted or twisted without this one. It is not so critical what the deeper or surer place is, but it is critical that it take you beyond a constricted fixation on dominance power or a readiness to be drawn into a struggle for such power. Without this "other place" to stand, you can easily be drawn into the strangest of processes and only later learn that you were sparring over power.

It might be helpful for you to have a few examples of some of the surer or deeper places I've learned about. It makes sense to me to negotiate in academic environments about what is best for students, what meets the university mission, what fulfills our philosophy of teaching, what provides knowledge to the larger society in a usable and meaningful fashion. It makes sense to me to negotiate in health care agencies for what benefits or heals our patients, what creates a healing environment for patients and their families, what heals communities suffering from a wide range of health deterrents, what leads to creative health promotion programs. It makes sense to me as a person to negotiate for the opportunity to grow and flourish, to love well, to preserve my integrity, to serve others, and to live out my own sense of the truth. I'm not selling any of these, just showing you how easy it is to find and articulate surer and deeper once you decide to do so.

An Exercise

You too will want to develop a list like the one above. Start this on a fresh page of your journal. Write down places where you think you customarily negotiate. Beside each one, write down at least one hope, dream, wish, or conviction you embrace that takes you beyond the simple goal of controlling the negotiation. See how broad in scope it is, how deep it takes you into the best of your personal character, how sure you are of its compelling quality for all humans. Isn't it amazing how painless this is!

Now write down all the reasons you can think of why you couldn't possibly introduce these surer and deeper issues into any of your negotiations. It is important to be honest and rigorous here. Don't censor anything. If it was easy, you'd probably be doing it already. You're not a dolt! There are risks; name them. Reflect on this a bit.

Now, select the absolutely easiest one and try it out the next time you have a chance. Don't ask a lot of yourself, just try one sentence early in the process. "Well, I think the important thing for us to all keep on the table is treating our customers the way we ourselves would like to be treated; we already have proof that this is profitable." Or "I think the really important thing to me is that you and this relationship are very dear and I hope you feel the same way about me; I want that to be the basis for your decision."

See what happens. Do it under optimal conditions; make sure you feel safe; see how it feels. Record your reaction in your journal. This is an exercise in creating an alternate reality. After a while, it gets really fun and you start feeling like Beethoven or Monet or Baryshnikov and want people to give you creativity awards. Even if you only do it where it is easy, you are doing your part to create a better negotiation than the idiocy of jockeying over power packets for the rest of your life. Isn't it amazing that you never tried this before?

It is important, I think, to learn this gradually, to start with easy and successful efforts, to simply test thinking larger rather than smaller. One of the ways we avoid surer and deeper is by testing the worst-case scenario, failing, and then excusing ourselves forever with cynical one-liners. Hence, set a goal to do one smashing success a week, then two a week, and work your way up to the tough ones. Eventually, it becomes a habit of sorts, like manipulation used to be in your life.

One last observation is noteworthy. All persons have unique stories within themselves about what is surer and deeper. This may be a philosophy of life, a value framework, a religious belief, a system of personal ethics or spirituality, or a cultural way of life. If it is dear to me, I may want it to suddenly be dear to you. One can be seduced into proselytizing. Not everyone agrees with everyone else's list. If you are trying to move beyond power negotiations to surer and deeper places, make sure that the surer and deeper places aren't ones others reject. Then you will simply find yourself having a new power struggle over the acceptability of your surer and deeper places.

I have a personal system of ethics and spirituality that is deeply important to me. I share it on occasion with others, but I never assume anyone at a negotiation shares it or wants to hear about it. This is not the starting point for surer and deeper. The starting point is shared values, common commitments to surer and deeper that we have all at some point claimed as our own. It is the Constitution and the Bill of Rights; civil rights; the mission of our schools, universities, hospitals, and businesses; the promises we make to one another. These shared values can take both me and all those with me at a table back to some more compelling time and place where we made those commitments and knew that we shared those beliefs. The deeper and surer, the more creative the outcome.

Tom Robbins (1990), in *Skinny Legs and All*, describes a dance of the seven veils where each veil, falling, reveals increasingly powerful truths. The last veil reveals that "everybody's got to figure it out for themselves" (p. 412). His insight removes the illusion that you can get somebody else to do it for you. This demonstrates that ways of being are not end points or finished products, but processes continuously unveiling new paradoxes of wisdom.

18

Way of Being Number Two

Be a Truth Teller

Recommending to others that they be truth tellers is pretty presumptuous, I think. It implies I think I know the truth or that you know the truth. I've already acknowledged that the only truth I can really offer is my little chunk of it, the often-limited and imperfect window on some larger sense of the truth that I have managed to struggle toward over time. But, limited and imperfect, it is my truth, and it is the stuff I have to work with when I seat myself at an uneven table. I have also discovered that while I may not be able to reveal some comprehensive sense of ultimate truth, I can recognize an untruth when it comes loping up and tries to sit on my lap or crawl in my brain. Often telling the truth involves saying where it isn't.

I have also discovered that if I am willing to tell the truth, imperfect as it is, this often frees others to reveal their particular window on the truth, and as others do this, we seem to all collectively get close to some expression of the truth. Each new window widens mine, and I grow. I do need to be ready to let the growth occur, and it will often alter my first insight considerably, but the final vision is always larger, richer, and more fulfilling. I have found that this readiness is essential, however, and when I get hooked on being right or having the whole truth, I fail to achieve this way of being, often becoming destructive and ineffective. This is to say that this is a pretty difficult way of being, but it has great promise in the long run. Being a truth teller enables it in others, and the truthfulness of the negotiations is increased. This also helps others acknowledge untruth.

Unevenness that is unacknowledged is in itself the first substantial untruth that is present at most uneven tables. Knowing and naming it early without rancor or self-pity is important. This needs to happen early so that those at the table realize you are there knowing this truth. Mentioning it halfway through the negotiations leaves others feeling tricked and manipulated, especially if you're able to demonstrate it is true. Sometimes I've found, however, that I'm not sure at first. I try to require myself to be sure. Then I acknowledge it. I also find I have to report then that I wasn't sure at first, but now I am, and why. This lends clarity and prevents others from feeling blindsided.

Becoming Truthful About Truth Telling

Being a truth teller is more difficult and complex than it looks at first blush. One must know the difference between telling the truth and bludgeoning people with it. I have made this error often enough that many people have taken the time to educate me about it, sometimes by bludgeoning me with that truth. You also have to know that your personal window on the truth is only one of a myriad of windows on truth. Hence, while it is of great value to tell people that you believe you are sitting at an uneven table, and why you perceive this, this does not make this their reality nor will your telling them ensure that they will see it as you do. Often I find that the initial response is more defensive than acknowledging, even when I am not bludgeoning, simply because acceptance of some uneven tables as "normal" is so common. Sometimes the statement is more confusing than clarifying to others if it introduces an insight into injustice that until that moment seemed merely the nature of things, sort of like deciduous trees losing leaves in the fall.

A Story

Negotiating for budgets for nursing initiatives, schools, programs, and projects has been for me one of the most fascinating and sometimes irritating processes of my career. A good deal of lip service is usually given to the positive feelings everyone has for nurses, what good women and men they are, how important they are, and what wonderful things they do. Then you look at the budget.

When you try to get good salaries for nurses or nurse educators, you are told that this will drive up the cost of health care, even though nurses can easily demonstrate that physicians earn up to ten times the average nursing salary. A national shortage of faculty in business and engineering has led to a competition among institutions to attract faculty. This involves better salaries and better benefit packages. This has not happened in nursing, and the shortage in nursing is more severe and will worsen steadily over the next thirty years.

When you try to get adequate resources for funding clinics and nursing care centers, you are told money is scarce, even though you know that hospitals are enormous fiscal operations. I started an inner-city clinic with less money than an average hospitalization cost in the United States. When you try to get money for educational programs or research projects, you are assured that even if you have an excellent proposal, nine or ten proposals will go unfunded for each one you get funded. In 1992 the federal government subsidized physician residency training programs in teaching hospitals—graduate medical education—at approximately $5.2 billion (Aiken & Sage, 1993, p. 191). During this same year, only 14 million federal dollars were invested in grants to training programs in nurse practitioner and nurse midwifery programs, despite shortages of personnel in each of these advanced-practice nursing fields (p. 209). It is hard to look casual while you face such inequities.

Recently, I tried to explain this to a colleague unfamiliar with the issues. One need not even struggle with vague generalities; all one needs to do is compare budgets, square footage, student-faculty ratio, research resources, educational opportunities, and job perks between medical faculty and nursing faculty to grasp the systematic inequity. These for me are the kind of "truths" that often come unwelcomed to an uneven table. My favorite image of this is a sense that my efforts at responsible professional negotiation are often responded to as if I am asking dad for a new dress for the senior prom and he frowns at me and says, "What's wrong with that nice pink one you wore for your eighth-grade graduation?"

My experience is that men who are accustomed to living their private lives generating and controlling resources for women to expend, and who feel secretly that these expenditures need control and supervision, can never quite negotiate a budget with a woman without this life pattern emerging. I sometimes feel like I am watching an instant replay of their latest conversation with a wife or daughter, or a script taught them by their fathers. Their ability to see this often is limited because to unveil this fact is to put their entire fiscal life patterning into question. While I can feel compassion for them, it doesn't improve my budget much.

This story reveals some of the challenges implicit in trying to be a truth teller. All of these facts about fiscal injustice relative to professional nursing are quite compelling. They are hard to alter since the magnitude of inequity is so severe. The truths you tell can have such substance that to address them requires immense changes. In addition, the facts can be interpreted in a variety of ways. One person might read these facts and say that nurses are a cheaper commodity and less valuable. Another would say that nurses are being exploited; this is an injustice and must be addressed. A third might say that they're wonderful "women" but they simply don't understand the world of finance and lack good judgment; obviously, we need to make these determinations for them since they are unable to do so wisely on their own behalf. My sense of what these facts mean may not coincide with anyone else's at the table.

You actually have to start from the premise that your truth is partial, ambiguous, tentative, and tainted. This is pretty hard to accept, since most of us want our truth to prevail and be declared total and immortal. Once you can own the limits of your own truth, however, you can request the same courtesy of others. Then, you are free to propose pooling many perspectives to get closer to some more vital expression of truth. This to me has always seemed a better way to solve the dilemma of the six blind men who described the elephant six ways because they all felt different parts of the elephant's body. Even as a child, I couldn't figure out why someone didn't suggest that all six blind men could have pooled their information to get a better idea of what an elephant was. No one ever suggested that to me.

I wish they had. It has taken me a long time to learn how to tell my truth clearly, knowing it is only partial but still of value, not in need of defending. It has taken me even longer to learn how to let it grow, alter, expand, and enrich itself by letting it be influenced by the truth others bring to the table. The helpless child never tells her truth; the omnipotent child wants her truth to prevail. Neither works well. Being firm but patient with these two kids fatigues me some days, but is the only way to increase the creative possibilities that emerge if I become a truth teller and support that in others.

Listening as a Catalyst to Creativity

If you wish to be a truth teller, you need to learn to listen to people closely. This first creates a norm for understanding their perception of the truth of a situation. You can also find where your truth and theirs concur and overlap. This is true to some degree with everyone. Then, when you want to tell your truth, you can indicate the ways in which you have common ground, rather than creating a sense that there is none, but only room for conflict. This is a learned skill, and it takes practice.

You can also begin to see where you do not overlap. This often is the place where I grow and learn. If I can turn down the volume of my own defensiveness, my need to be right, my need to prevail, I can often learn a great deal from these moments. Often I fail, but when I succeed, it is well worth the effort. These places of difference are where the creative new idea emerges, if I let it do so.

A Story

I had a Kellogg Leadership Fellowship for three years, one that gave me a virtual smorgasbord of wonderful learning and relating opportunities. Early in the fellowship, I decided to go to Cuernavaca, Mexico, to study Spanish in an immersion program. It involved living with a Mexican family for sixteen days and only speaking Spanish. We were not only invited to learn the language but also the culture. It was a wonderful and challenging experience.

Early in the process, I realized I was feeling strong reactions to all the brilliant colors everywhere. Cuernavaca has a very steady climate, with an annual temperature range of about ten degrees, moderate and pleasant at all times. The blooming flowers everywhere seemed riotous. The culture seemed to me to reflect the flowers everywhere. People wore vivid fresh colors; the painted walls, decor, and murals were dazzling; the entire environment teemed with gay sparkling hues of every band of the rainbow.

I suddenly realized that I was a German-American and specialized in fourteen variants of monochromatic neutrals. I almost fell asleep looking at my wardrobe. I realized I thought it made me look serious, that it was safe, nonexuberant, even guarded. This gave me pause. I began to understand why we need one another. Only a Mexican, I decided, could save me from my hapless rigidities about color.

Placing myself in the hands of my host and hostess, I went experimenting and exploring. They laughed warmly at my caution and patiently watched me imagine all this color in my life. Slowly I grew in comfort, and began to realize how enriched my life was becoming with all this color. I discovered that somewhere in me, my passion for rainbows, which I had since childhood, could be reactivated if I let those with the ease, wisdom, and comfort with the process serve as my teachers. They helped me make some purchases to take home, to visit some sites where color could properly overwhelm me. I think we all grew from the experience. But because they had a window on the truth that I needed to learn, I needed to listen to their lessons.

If you listen well, you also set a norm at the table for listening well. If you can begin to identify what others have said reflectively, they sense the value of being listened to and may decide that you too could be worth listening to. Most of us most of the time prepare a retort while we listen. I have found over time that when I do this I miss so much of what others are saying that my retort is highly inappropriate and merely indicates that I failed to listen actively to what was actually being said. This gives others the option then of choosing not to listen to me.

Truth Telling as a Measure of Self-Honesty

There are some truth tests you need when you want to be a truth teller. If your truth is an obsession, it is not truth. If your truth harms or belittles others, it is not truth. If your truth aims to diminish others, it is not truth. These are all attacking behaviors posing as the truth. They are pseudotruths and should not be mistaken for an effort at "truth" telling. It has become so commonplace to use truth destructively, even as a way of exercising dominance power, that even if your truth passes all these tests, it may be perceived as an obsession that harms, belittles, and diminishes others. We have made it acceptable in our culture to use truth to do injury. As a result, for some people all truth not like their own feels like an effort to harm.

Thus, the touchstone for these tests needs to be the rigor of your own self-honesty, not the responses of others. Sometimes an unwelcome truth is denied credibility by noting that it hurts others. This is another variant on manipulation. The fact that a truth is disturbing does not make it untrue or harmful. The fact that it upsets people may indeed indicate how close it is to reality, and how much denial nestles in the heart and mind of the reactive person. I know that this is often true of me, and the truths that have taught me the most I often first experience as threats—insights that I try hard to deny or to defend against. Many of the world's great injustices were truths unstated lest they hurt someone. Hurt is sometimes a defense to avoid self-responsibility.

I may also confuse truth telling with indiscriminate superficial commentaries on everything and everyone. This is merely mental laziness or self-aggrandizement, an effort to draw attention to myself or evoke admiration or involvement from others. It evokes a relationship predicated on insistence, on noticing my presence. I can thus use my candor to meet other unstated goals, while trying to give the appearance of being a truth teller. This too is another touchstone for truth telling. As becomes apparent, the motive of the truth teller is a critical factor. Being unaware of my own motives merely makes me dangerous, not innocent.

Unveiling Truths

Truths unrelated to the issues on the table have limited utility and may simply serve as distractions or avoidance maneuvers. The truths that enable conflict identification and conflict resolution are the truths one brings to a table, and not others. Among these, however, there are often truths that are ignored or denied. Putting these on the table can lead to a mixed reception, often at the same table. It has been my experience that many people are relieved that the real issues are on the table. Often, however, one or another person is upset, even outraged, having assumed that the issue being avoided would never foolishly be raised by anyone. It is my experience that both racism and sexism are often dealt with in this fashion at many uneven tables.

This often unveils a covert dominance negotiation: I control what is on the table and that way I control the outcome; there are certain things that we will ignore so I can stay in power. This kind of covert issue is not uncommon, and it takes both awareness and courage to attend to it. Often the table is uneven precisely because some truth is unacknowledged. Confronting this can be discomforting; ignoring it makes you party to a dishonest negotiation. You need to be prepared to grow from the role of truth teller. If you do it well, you cannot avoid growth. It will greet you at every turn. It is helpful to remember that at many tables, some truth wasn't there because it wasn't invited. The fact that you bring it forward may often simply seem like recalcitrance, neglect of the unspoken rules, bad taste, or rebelliousness. You need to be prepared for these possibilities, since they can lead to active discounting of what you have to say. You also have to make sure that you are not merely engaging in recalcitrance and rebelliousness posing as truth telling.

It perhaps seems too obvious to say so, but being a truth teller is actually a pretty risky business. It is not an accident that they have created whistleblower protection legislation. But being a truth teller can also be liberating and does encourage a good deal of self-honesty. You cannot really be a truth teller if you harbor a whole bevy of self-deceptions on the side. These become the best way to discredit you. Hiding them doesn't work either, since they will out, one way or another. Better to just go for the truth, or you will never really be able to exercise this particular way of being. Finding your own truth, of course, is an endless process, so you will always be this way imperfectly, but you can choose to get better and better at it.

In my experience, a common way of discrediting an unwelcome truth is to tell me that my delivery was imperfect, too blunt, too indirect, too frequent, too seldom, too strident, too modest . . . there's a list here. I have learned over time that the best thing to do with this is just acknowledge that the delivery was doubtless quite imperfect, and then ask if this in any way mitigates or alters the truth of what was said. I know it doesn't, and so do others. I find I have to reflect on this issue, however, since I can easily get defensive about the imperfections of my delivery.

Being distracted by critical appraisals of delivery can keep you from telling the truth. Start with the assumption that you will say it imperfectly. If others cling to the delivery as an issue, it usually seems to me that they are actually saying that they simply didn't like the particular truth I presented. Knowing what the concern actually is can prove helpful in staying clear in your own mind, heart, and soul. That may actually be the next truth you are called on to face.

Over the years, I have learned that when I am sitting at an uneven table, many other people at the table who know the same truths as I do elect to sit back and let me do the truth telling on their behalf. There just aren't enough truth tellers around, and when folks find one, they like to ask for a lot of overtime. These are the people who meet you in the hall after the negotiation and say, "I really appreciated what you said in there; you're absolutely right!" Beware of such people. They are not truth tellers. Real truth tellers say that at the table.

If there are several persons at the table embracing this silent agreement, you may find yourself in a situation where many people at the table agree with you but sit mutely watching the negotiation as if attending an entertaining movie. It is important to note when this happens. Their silence signals that the possibilities at this table may be limited, that the negotiation cannot proceed openly. The inability of many at the table to support truth tellers warrants monitoring.

Supporting Other Truth Tellers

Actually, this is one of the most effective roles of a skillful truth teller: to accentuate and support the truth telling of others and do so publicly, at the table. This helps indicate to others at the table how widespread acknowledgment of a given truth actually is. There may even be a majority, or one may emerge. Asking others to concur or to differ also helps. This tends to make it clearer where the truth tellers are. It also helps the people at the table who are uncertain. They begin to see that more than one person is noticing something that they had failed to see or were too timid or fearful to acknowledge.

There is a rhythm to effective truth telling. One does not simply go in and shower people with buckets of exclamatory sentences. To be effective, truth telling needs to fit the flow of the discussion, the moments of openness, and the opportunities that emerge naturally. It weaves its way into the process without trumpets. It simply is, and creates its own power separate from the truth teller. To proceed in any other fashion is to diminish the power of the truth, to draw attention not to the truth but to oneself.

Every Voiced Penelope

Truth is my exacting lover,
love the energy. The work
is in the dark places; the
light grows if you choose.
The journey is arduous, but
as nothing, looking back,
from home. Housecleaning
continues, singing. I am the
music of the spheres. It is
my laughter you hear in the
night, flowing in your dreams.
I am calling you to the sweet
eternal frolic of the dance.
I am waiting for you here,
preparing an abundant banquet,
preparing a celebration,
coming home.

—pbk

As I noted at the outset of this part of the book, the ways of being actually are a gestalt, or field of action. Truth telling is intimately connected with inhabiting the deepest, surest human space. If truth telling is not well received at an uneven table, it is often because there is an implicit commitment to avoiding sure or deep human spaces. Truth telling tends to reveal that fact. This is important to reflect on, since it often is a key factor in the potential for manifesting the other ways of being.

An Exercise

This is a retrospective. You don't have to do anything tomorrow or next week, unless you decide to do so without my urging. For now, all you have to do is recall and reflect.

Recall a recent conflict you experienced, be it with a family member, a work colleague, an old friend, or a perfect stranger. Recall the conflict in as much detail as you can. Reflect on it a while. Now recall it again. Now reflect again. These old conflicts aren't all that fun to revisit, but that's the task for the moment.

In your journal, try to briefly write down the key details as you recall them. Now record, as precisely as you can, what you believe the conflict was about. Next record, as precisely as you can, what you assume the other person thought the conflict was about. Doing this carefully is worth the trouble, so take your time.

Now, study those two ideas for a while and see if there is something more substantial underneath each of your fundamental positions. Try out some ideas. Was the conflict, for either of you, really about vanity, or greed, or fear, or shame, or the horror of making an error, or the loss of face in front of the other person? Did one of you want to get the other one to think a certain way, so both of you would think the same way? Was there something one of you thought was the real issue but neither of you would state? Did one of you want to get even? What was underneath this conflict?

If you're real honest with yourself, you'll find something, usually for both of you. If you repeat this question of "What was really going on?" several times, you will find you can get closer and closer to the real nature of the conflict as you actually experienced it. All conflict is ultimately inner conflict, inside the parties to the conflict. You always have direct access to your half, if you want to find it. Take the time to struggle with this for a while.

As you identify these underlying themes, write them down as candidly as you can. Just say them in simple terms, such as, "I really wanted him to say I actually had a very good idea, even if he didn't want to go along with it," or "I wanted her to tell me I'd done a good job, even if it wasn't perfect." Keep writing down these underlying issues until you are either fatigued by the effort or bored to tears from staring at this one lousy conflict.

Now, go through your list of underlying themes. Imagine each as a "truth" that you might have "told" at some point in the conflict. Beside each, write down whether or not you would have been willing to tell the other party this truth. Don't just imagine or theorize; actually write a yes or a no. Study these answers.

Determine the degree to which the list about the other party involves either projection or blaming. Put a large "X" by all these. They are of limited utility, beyond informing you of your ability to participate in the most popular American sport—projection and blaming. The fact that you are doing this is often the reason you can't say your truths, of course. You may simply be too caught up in the projection or too guilty about the blaming. The list about the other person is interesting only in that it tells you what you thought was occurring. You probably don't really know what was occurring for others unless you can borrow their journals when they read this book and see what they wrote.

The underlying themes you wrote about yourself, however, are your truths to struggle with. Whether the other person knows these or not, whether you were willing to share them or not, they persist as the things you believed to be true. The fact that they were not shared is significant, of course, if you're interested in becoming a truth teller.

This is a useful diagnostic on the role of conscious truth telling in a conflict. It is also a model for learning. Every time you have a conflict, instead of ruminating about it, pouting about it, seeking revenge, or blotting it out of your brain, try this exercise. You will quickly discover the role of truth telling in your conflicts. You will also unveil new choices.

Because I am an open-minded person about this issue, I am willing to let you use this very same journal to keep a record of these conflicts and the truth components you find in them. This is of course very generous on my part, and eliminates for you at least one excuse for failing to follow through on your next conflict: asking yourself the tough question of whether or not you elect to be a truth teller.

19

Way of Being Number Three
Honor Your Integrity, Even at Great Cost

It's actually pretty hard to find someone who would publicly announce that selling your soul is wise or clever, that short-changing your character is visionary, or that losing your integrity is of no real significance. Integrity is a bit like parenthood; there's a great deal of agreement on its importance and an equal degree of indifference to assuring its soundness and excellence. We in the United States, often too eager for the fast fix, the quick-and-dirty solution, the superficial reassurance, are loath to grapple with the complexity and struggle that honoring our integrity may ask of us. The neglect of personal integrity may be the single most powerful explanation for both our cynicism and our greed. We want a lot without paying the price.

Thus, this way of being may sound quite acceptable, and would rarely evoke overt opposition, yet it demands a great deal of us. At an uneven table, it may only be honored at great cost. The most fundamental reason for this is quite simply that if the table was set unevenly to start with, somewhere someone has already decided to ignore or deny inequity and hopes you will, too. If you refuse, there will very likely be a price to pay.

Or in some cases, people set the table unevenly, acknowledge this to you, and then wish you well, sort of like sending Daniel into the lion's den. Sometimes I have sensed that the table has actually been set so the inequity can be addressed without being resolved.

Once Daniel is eaten alive, no more Daniel, no more problem. This is important to be aware of, since it clearly is a sophisticated version of dominance power at its worst: a person with power has the control to set the table, invites me to it knowing I am disadvantaged, and then watches the show. Such people try to claim they are proponents of justice. Be wary with them!

Over time, I have learned the wisdom of this wariness. If these persons were proponents of justice, they would clearly communicate all these covert assumptions and be truth tellers themselves. If you invite someone to the table under conditions of inequity, you need to be prepared to acknowledge that fact and deal with it without harms to people at the table. Seeing if I sink or swim may amuse or entertain others, but it does not resolve conflict. I am particularly susceptible to this manipulation, because I don't sink readily. I rather stupidly start thrashing about, trying to stay afloat. Participating in such a charade is really just one more version of an invitation to sell my integrity. It took me a long time to realize this, so if you too struggle with it, you have my empathy.

Assuming Moral Agency

The most common challenge to my integrity as a person at an uneven table has been the assumption that I am not a moral agent. Since I am a woman and a nurse, the cultural beliefs that lead to that assumption have captured my attention. It has taken me some time to realize that just because I think I am an independent and adult moral agent, this does not lead to others supporting my conviction. More often, the assumption is made that I am incapable of or unlikely to exercise moral agency, and hence moral choosing will or must be made on my behalf.

When I first began to experience this, I was very confused by it. I knew their belief was not valid, but I couldn't figure out why others thought it was. That's how I found out the really insidious dimensions of Greco-Roman democracy and the roots of Western philosophy. The idea of "man" as a rational animal has tended to emphasize rationality and traditionally has only encompassed males. Women have been seen as less than rational and less than men. I actually felt that they assigned to me the animal part of the equation, as in "and with women we express our animality." This hunch is truer than most men and women want to acknowledge.

Hence, moral decision making grounded in principled rationality was the purview of men and beyond my competence as a woman. The fact that my moral agency has often addressed not only rationality but also the relational and receptive dimensions of human nature simply worsened the situation. I was declared irrational, emotionally subjective, and unscientific. How could I ever be trusted to independently identify the good and choose it over the evil? Clearly, others would have to make these choices for me and impose them on me if necessary.

It took me many years to realize that when I refused to accept this interpretation of my reality, the refusal proved my moral inadequacy. I failed to see and embrace the good as defined for me. Then I proved myself rebellious and confused, unwilling to comply and submit. It was no wonder I needed all that dominance power to keep me in line, to keep me from doing rash and foolish things, emotionally charged and bereft of rational virtue as I was. I often became a naïve accomplice in this process, rebelling in my insecurity or withdrawing out of uncertainty. It has taken me many years to fully understand this dynamic. It is often so subtle that it is difficult to name and comprehend. It is so insulting that it is easy to become cruel and destructive in response to it. It is so pervasive that it is hard to sustain your own sense of reality when everyone else assumes another reality. The national dialogue on biomedical ethics provides a useful exemplar of this strange process of denied moral agency. A principle-based ethical system, it rarely includes reflections on the patient-advocacy-based ethics developed and supported by nurse scholars and ethicists, and in several cases written into state nursing practice law. Rather, it is assumed that "experts" will resolve health care ethical dilemmas according to a set of applied principles, and nurses will be expected not only to accept these resolutions but also to take specific patient care actions based on them. Often the decision maker has little direct experience with patient care or little understanding of the power of the relationship between patient and nurse.

Palliative care or end of life decisions are useful examples in this regard. While the nurse is usually the person most present and available to patients, and best equipped to observe them, and their families over time, the information nurses offer concerning patients' wishes is often dismissed as irrelevant, or merely the "emotional" observations of a nurse "too close" to the family. Relationship-based ethics are discounted, as is the moral agency of the nurse. What is more disturbing is the assumption that the nurse will give care guided by another's moral choice, or fail to exercise moral agency when others neglect patients' rights and well-being.

A Story

During the past few years I have had the opportunity to watch closely the experiences of a young nurse who sued her hospital under whistleblower provisions of the state's nurse practice act. She had challenged the neglect of patients' rights to refuse care, and had subsequently experienced retaliatory behavior from the hospital. Her right to moral agency was not only ignored, it was actively denied and viewed as an inappropriate questioning of physician decision making.

The judge, who had strong affiliations with some of the involved hospital physicians, had not recused himself in this case. As the case unfolded, he publicly expressed surprise when he learned that the state's nurse practice act required this nurse to take the action she had taken. He also repeatedly denied the jury access to information and testimony that would have demonstrated how seriously the rights of patients had actually been compromised, and the resultant damages to them and their families.

Although a jury found in the nurse's favor, the fundamental assumptions of the hospital did not change. In addition, the hospital's defense team structured their case so that the nurse manager, who had participated in the retaliation, was held culpable, but the physician who required the retaliation was held harmless. Because this was a state hospital, the hospital lawyers were actually state district attorney officers. This created the anomalous situation of patient rights, defended by the nurse, being opposed by the state in order to protect its hospital and its physician.

Discussing the outcome of the case with the jury forewoman, I was struck by her observation. The jury, she noted, wondered where all the other nurses were who also should have challenged this neglect of patients' rights. Why, they wondered, was this nurse left to stand alone when so many knew of the problems? They were not only observable by the hospital staff involved, but had been documented by several patients in a variety of public arenas.

The answers, of course, were instructive. Some nurses had taken a comparable moral stance and had been actively blackballed from employment at the hospital, their careers irreparably damaged. During the court proceedings, these nurses came forth to stand by this nurse, but few others did. The nursing leadership of both the hospital and its affiliated school of nursing gave veiled directives advising that nurses should not be present in court to support the nurse plaintiff, in effect supporting those who harmed the nurse, and substantiating the concern about further retaliation.

The nurse was understandably hurt by this lack of support, particularly when it included the nursing faculty who had taught her that she was obligated to take the action she took. Those nurses who did stand by her understood that in doing so, they too risked retaliation. They knew that rather than being admired by their peers, they too would be labeled as "troublemakers." Only the jury it seemed, understood this nurse's courageous moral agency and respected it.

The social construction in this institution is thus demonstrable. Nurses are not viewed as moral agents. Hence, when a physician engages in an unethical practice, it is assumed that the nurse cannot and will not challenge this, but will simply do as she or he is told. Perhaps more distressing, many nurses concur. Social constructions of reality have powerful implications.

The lack of comprehension of this issue is profound and is most easily evidenced by the systematic bias reflected in the discussion of these issues, even in such outstanding resources as the Hastings Center, where discourse about health care ethics frequently simply ignores the presence and power of the nurse as a moral agent. Patients do not do this; they count on our moral agency, our advocacy on their behalf. They also share with us concerns they may share with no one else; we are there to hear them. This information influences our moral judgments.

Hence, someone else determining, on my behalf, that some action is acceptable does not make it acceptable to me, or to my patients. To assume so is to assume that I am not a moral agent, or that my moral agency is inferior to the "superior" persons who made the judgment. The tainting of ethics with unconscious dominance power concerns can influence decisions about integrity for just about everyone.

These issues have proven useful to me in grasping the nature of this way of being. If someone determines I am not a moral agent, that in itself is disturbing. If someone determines that they must make moral choices on my behalf, as if I were unable to do so, that is more disturbing. That they would actually ask me to enact their moral choice, however, is the most disturbing dimension of the lot. And this happens all the time for any person in our culture viewed as unequal, inferior, or in need of dominance power control. The implicit assumption is that the person exercising dominant power is better equipped to make moral choices and may have to impose them.

Avoiding Moral Agency

It is important here to note this is in part a sustainable model because many people don't want to exercise moral agency, would prefer that someone else do so on their behalf, and then carry out

another's directives as if they somehow were assured of righteousness. We who are of German ancestry have deep memories of the
implications of that rationale. Hitler was wrong.

Unfortunately, in many world religions, the same assumptions
are made: "superior" persons can or should determine moral agency
for others. The call is to obedience, and the willingness of "superior" persons to acknowledge their human limits is itself often limited. They may tell me something is God's will for me, and if I
believe them, I find myself carrying out their wishes, invariably
tainted with human imperfection, in the hope that God's will is
now being done.

Over time, I have learned that many people are strikingly unable
to distinguish between patriarchal dominance control and moral
agency. Many persons assume these are the same thing, both those
controlling and those being controlled. Where such confusion prevails, my choice to exercise moral agency can be risky, particularly
when my choices may differ from those imposed on me by others
who believe they control me. To hope to draw these others into an
honest exploration of an alternative understanding of the situation
is even more demanding, and sometimes more dangerous.

Being Willing to Stand Alone

What has become clear to me is that I usually have to take full
responsibility for explaining my understanding of my own moral
agency. I rarely find that it is assumed at an uneven table. I also find
that once I do so, others may not be willing to support or endorse
my decision. This lack of support and endorsement emerges both
from those who believed they would be my moral agent and from
those who have elected to let someone else be theirs. It is one of
the times at an uneven table when you can really feel alone if you
are trying to manifest these ways of being.

I would actually like to be more encouraging about all this, but
moral agency is not one of our country's current strong suits, and

we are ill-advised to assume otherwise. The sudden flurry of ethics committees for all manner of things has itself become a tool to discredit others politically, and conversely, to claim a moral soundness when absolved of suspected breaches of ethics. Crisp, spare, lucid ethical clarity is in short supply. We would not have become so enamored of cynicism if the situation were otherwise.

In addition, if you go to the table knowing that you will honor your integrity, the various unacknowledged invitations to turn over your moral agency to another person will capture your attention. You will notice these invitations. You will become sensitized to the assumption that this is acceptable to you. You will begin to clarify for yourself your own moral boundaries and see when others wish to encroach on them, even if naïvely or unconsciously. You will also notice when others ask you to turn over your moral agency with the promise of a reward for doing so, or a punishment for failing to do so.

Actually, the clarification is powerful in itself. The struggle to reach such clarity helped me finally understand how often my conflicts with others reduced to the simple assumption that I was not a moral agent, or could not exercise moral agency, or did not choose to do so. My lack of clarity was my responsibility, of course, and helped me better comprehend the ways I could shortchange my own integrity by simplistic trust, careless neglect, lack of discrimination, cowardice, or laziness. These problems of integrity are mine to own, and I have learned over time to do so more deliberately. This is one of the ways of being at uneven tables that has proven enriching to me. I see it retrospectively as an advantage of some substance.

alone

for once, finally, this bridge i built
and cross on over, over again
on my bridge, my blood bones bridge
i built of my hard fibrous womb.

i birthed this truth, labored sharp,
incessantly, obsessed, compelled;
forced forth these wisdoms alone
in some dark squat of valor.

i wrote this trembling song
to celebrate this ragged victory
that i still half distrust:
crossing over, birthing, alone.

　　—pbk

Balancing

The clarity gained has been worth the struggle for me. The clarity also, however, has resulted in a second, more complex set of dynamics that are a part of this way of being at an uneven table. Earlier in this section of the book I drew a picture of emerging and dominant paradigms as I experience them. Integrity is a dimension embedded in each. For persons who view the dominant paradigm as the only—or at least the superior—vision of reality, the guidelines for moral choice often emerge as predictable, rational, logical principles of action. For persons who view the emerging paradigm as the only or at least the superior vision of reality, guidelines for moral choice often emerge as relational, contexted, intuitive ways of responding. Both of these persons can be found at the uneven tables you visit, trying to make sense of personal integrity.

As you know by now, I am interested in the balance between these two paradigms, the desire to find the rhythmic interchange, honoring the possibilities and strengths of each, the synergistic possibilities. As such, I craft a vision of personal integrity acceptable to neither group. This does not increase my sense of gaining support and enthusiasm for my exercise of personal integrity. The polarity created by these divergent views, and others, complicates the effort to honor one's personal integrity. It is clearly a choice I must make in a spirit of deep self-responsibility, and I have to learn to accept the fact that it may make sense to no one but myself.

This all seems to say, of course, that honoring your integrity inevitably costs a great deal. This is not necessarily so, in my experience, however. I have found that the struggle to do so openly and clearly tends to introduce moral integrity into the negotiation. I didn't really mean to do this, actually. I started out just trying to say that I was indeed a moral agent, no matter who thought I was not, and that my exercise of moral agency was mine to determine, even if it concurred with no one else's judgments. I think I began doing it defensively at best, to try to explain that I wasn't trying to keep the conflict going, I just couldn't go along with some of the assumptions popular at most uneven tables.

What I discovered, inadvertently, was that honoring my integrity had gotten to be a pretty large issue for me, evoking a good deal of my personal strength and energy. In the process, I had introduced the focus of personal integrity, and others, almost with a sigh of relief, joined me in supporting the premise of my stance. They did not necessarily make the same choices as I made, but they did concur with the importance of personal integrity, and thus moved the negotiation, with me, to a surer deeper place with more substantive levels of truth telling.

Over time, I have learned that clearly articulating and supporting my own personal integrity lends credibility to my efforts and gives both me and others the option of exercising moral persuasion as a dimension of a negotiation. Because one can also assume such a position cynically or manipulatively, the position is of course rightly tested. I have some sympathy with people who do the testing, since they too are no doubt weary of the cynicism that saps the life energy of us all. Some tests are themselves actually cynical, however, and come as invitations to cut deals that compromise your integrity—sort of like dirty tricks to deflect the negotiation from a surer and deeper place. As a physician colleague said to me once when he was threatening to eliminate me from a collaborative effort that I was deeply committed to, "Perhaps you won't be able to compromise enough to participate." When messages of this nature are sent, it is helpful to remember that this may be the "last line of defense" against moral power and the inclusion of moral agency in a negotiation.

Finding Courage

I find this particular way of being at an uneven table really challenging. In trying to determine why it is so difficult, I've had to face my own lack of courage. I know I want a larger group with me in the effort, that I don't much like being so alone with this way of being. There is little cultural support for this dimension of being a full human. It is more socially acceptable, in my experience, to simply be silent, particularly, it seems, for women. Perhaps because there is so much cynicism about moral conduct, so much dishonesty about ethics as a political charade, it is difficult to publicly announce personal integrity as a human value. It is also scary, because then all sorts of people who want to discredit you start searching for your moral failures.

I personally have had enough moments in my history where I lacked wisdom and courage, when I couldn't find the path to the right outcome, that I share this sense of vulnerability. I know that if persons want to discover something about me that proves I am morally imperfect, they can do so. I believe this can actually be done about everyone. This vulnerability is often used to silence people. This will not necessarily increase your comfort level at an uneven table, but it does have to be faced if you want to embrace this way of being.

So, you just have to go ahead and risk it. You have to honor your personal integrity even though others may try to discredit you by showing that you are morally imperfect. It helps to admit this at the outset, to acknowledge that you're imperfect but that it hasn't stopped you from still trying to honor your integrity as best you can, whenever you can. This may help decrease the anxiety that bubbles up when someone at an uneven table, eager to eliminate moral conduct as a dimension of the negotiation, points out your moral failures. It is helpful for me to remember that they must have some reason for wanting to keep personal integrity out of the negotiation.

Most people, in my experience, actually welcome the opportunity to begin to focus on personal integrity as part of a negotiation. Most people like to have the best in themselves drawn forth, not the worst. Most people would really like to be more of who they are when they are the person they like a lot. Introducing moral choice gives them access to that person in themselves and changes the negotiation quite dramatically. While some people will persist in wanting to sacrifice their own or another's integrity, saying that they are more "realistic," coping with such people is a modest price to pay if all the other people at an uneven table are trying to reach for the best in themselves. It is a difficult way of being, but an intensely rewarding one. It can, of course, also dramatically alter outcomes in any negotiation, since it moves the process to a focus on more profound and compelling human issues and adds strength to truth telling.

An Exercise

This exercise can give you an opportunity to determine the ways you tend to honor and not honor your integrity. I thought I'd tell you that at the outset, so you can start alternately being proud of yourself and being remorseful. I've tried to tell you that I think this one is difficult. You don't want some wimpy exercise that avoids that fact, do you?

Once more, this exercise asks you to be reflective. Think back over the last few weeks to any conflicts you have had. You will tend to recall those that were either very nice or very ugly in the end. They are still rattling around in your heart and soul, and you are still worrying about them anyway, so they must have been important. If you've had a nice conflict-free few weeks, I commend you. Then go back farther.

Briefly list these with a few key descriptors. The other party, the focus, and the outcome are enough, as in "my daughter Lisa, the car, stayed home." Now, beside each one put a plus for the ones where you liked the outcome and a minus for the ones where you didn't like the outcome. This shouldn't be too difficult. Since you could recall the conflict, you probably had strong feelings about it. If the outcome was mixed, you probably ultimately didn't like something about it or it wouldn't still be haunting you. Don't feel too bad if all of them are ones where you didn't like the outcome. These do haunt us more readily.

Now, recall each one for a while and reflect on it. Were there issues of personal integrity involved, for you or for the other person? What were they? How did you react to these? Did either of you state them? What happened when they were stated? If they weren't, do you think it could have made a difference? How? How would you have stated your issues of personal integrity? Would you have tried to get a need to control interpreted as an issue of personal integrity? How? Were these conflicts about winning and losing? Who won? Who lost? What was won? What was lost?

Do this for a while. This is actually a very difficult exercise. You may want to revisit it later, or a few times. These questions do not have easy answers. They do raise useful issues, however. These questions can actually be useful for the rest of your life!

Now, take a few moments and try to write five to ten sentences about the issues of personal integrity that are really important to you, that you believe you would never really feel good about compromising in any negotiation. Just write them in your own words; they're not going to be on the national news tonight. Think about them a while. Does anyone know about these other than you? Would you be able or willing to share them with others during a conflict? Could you do so without anger or defensiveness? What role does personal integrity play in your negotiations with others around conflict? If there is no role, why is this? Do you like it that way? What choices do you have, and what choices will you make about all of this? Did you know the choices could make a difference?

———————

20

Way of Being Number Four
Find a Place for Compassion at the Table

Negotiation is ultimately a very human process. It is transacted among vulnerable and limited humans, all of whom harbor their personal set of needs, hopes, dreams, fears, fantasies, vanities, failures, and faults. This is not so much bad news as true news, and the striking and even exciting thing is that we stumbling humans do so well at it, given the challenge. The ability to face this true news is the first step in finding a place for compassion at the table.

Becoming Clear About Compassion

Before you seat compassion, however, it is useful to make sure you understand just who you've invited to the table and why you've done so. The concept of compassion is central to many Eastern religions and philosophies but enjoys a less central role in the cultures of the West. Here it is often confused with pity, sentimentality, or superficial niceness. Compassion demands more. It is the capacity to be aware of distress and to wish to alleviate it, to bear with, to suffer with. When we feel it for others, it is reflected in our willingness to place ourselves in their reality as they experience it, to feel as they feel and to feel with them. In such feeling, I wish the other well, relief from the distress. I stand ready to manifest that wish. Compassion assumes empathic oneness with others.

Compassion is most often confused with pity. In pity I stand outside others, I do not join them in their humanness but observe it as an outsider. I may, and often do, feel pity in a way that defines the other as less than myself. I may regret their sorrows or hardships, but I do not share these. They are not mine to feel or know. In our culture, pity thus often has a connotation of disdain, as if, in looking down on another, I elevate myself. This is perhaps inevitable in a culture enmeshed in a paradigm of power and hierarchical social structuring. Pity becomes the polite face for a secret disdain, a belief that someone else's distress can best be interpreted as my victory and their defeat over life's travails. I may even take a certain smug satisfaction in feeling pity. All this has tended to give pity a bad name, with good reason.

Sometimes a situation calls me to compassion, and the best I can muster is superficial niceness or sentimentality. Perhaps I don't really want to feel what others are feeling, to know and understand their pain. I may want to avoid the discomfort this creates, the confrontation with my own limited humanness. The lack of compassion in this culture for people with AIDS is an instructive example of distancing from pain I fear, do not understand, or experience as threatening. The further I drift from understanding my own vulnerability, the less I am able to experience and manifest compassion. In that light, it is perhaps equally instructive to witness the extraordinary compassion that many persons in the gay community are able to manifest for those members of their community who are either HIV infected or living with AIDS. Understanding vulnerability in myself assists me in feeling compassion for others.

Feeling Compassion for Myself

As is thus apparent, the first and most challenging place where I learn to manifest compassion is toward myself. Until I can honestly face my own limits and failures, I will tend to deny them, to run from them. In this country, we like to solve this dilemma by simply projecting them onto others and blaming others. It is a sloppy solution to fear, but a popular one nonetheless. Then, if I want to strike out or hate this vulnerability, I can hate it in others and avoid the tough confrontation with my own limits. To successfully break into my own self-indulgent drift toward projection and blaming, I need to first learn compassion toward myself. I personally have found this insight easier to grasp intellectually than to make real on an experiential and feeling level in my own life.

Compassion at an uneven table changes everything. If I am compassionate with myself, I forgive myself, without self-indulgence, for my failures and limits. I am then more able to give the same compassion to others, and therefore the same forgiveness, once more without indulgence. If I can make a commitment to trying to seat compassion at the table, I myself find the position I take changes. I enter the negotiation without demanding perfection of others or myself. I know before I start that I am going to forgive myself and others. This changes how I approach the entire process. In the end, it is liberating.

Honoring the Challenge of Compassion

To be compassionate and to forgive does not alter my commitment to finding a surer and deeper place, or being a truth teller, or honoring my personal integrity, but it takes the edge of harshness out of their manifestation and reminds me that all of us at the table are vulnerable and limited humans. Compassion is slow to anger, and thus my responses slow down. I am willing to reflect, to listen better, to try to understand. If I discover that it is difficult for me to keep compassion at the table, I know I need a time-out. I can usually tell this because my engine starts racing. I do not slow down; I do not reflect. This usually means that I am either losing touch with my compassion for myself or losing touch with my compassion for others.

Negotiations that can harm do occur. It is naïve and irresponsible to think otherwise. They can harm me and others. If I am harmed, I need to have enough compassion with myself to leave if this is wise, to give myself time to heal, and to stay away from tables that might further harm me until I am healed. If I do not take responsibility for this, I will probably go to tables needy, unable to experience compassion, and either invite more harm or inflict harm. With compassion, I discover that there are some tables that I should never go to or never return to.

Sometimes it is hard for me to find compassion, or I am unwilling to seat compassion at the table. "Any table but this one!" I say to myself. This is a clue. It does not mean that someone at the table deserves less compassion than others. It means that somewhere there is an unanswered question in me. Until I find that answer, this is a table I avoid. If I can't seat compassion at the table, I shouldn't be there. It is a simple guideline for me, but one that has proven invaluable.

I usually try to take the time to find out exactly why I am unable to seat compassion at the table. Sometimes the reason is fairly clear. No one else at the table wants to seat compassion, and I am at an uneven table. In such a situation, the table is not worth my time and energy, and there are better tables to go to. In other cases, some unacknowledged intolerance or vanity or fear lurks in my heart. My unwillingness to give up these little chunks of nastiness are the real issue. Then I have the option of facing these and growing from the confrontation. Such a process needs to occur before I go to the table, though. Waiting until I get there to have my clever insight is too late, and harms are often done if I neglect to follow my own guidelines. Doing my own hard shadow work becomes part of the path to effectiveness at an uneven table.

I was not born with an excess of patience. I have a high energy level, a capacity for quick comprehension, and an appreciation for the total symphony of life at full volume. These give me wonderful life experiences, but they do not help address an already serious deficiency in patience. Thus, my engine runs at high idle most of the time, and it has taken many years for me to slow it down enough to learn the patience that is the basis for compassion. I am not always successful, but I know the power of compassion when I am successful.

As I write this book, I sometimes feel my engine race ahead, and so I try to put the task aside and find a diversion. The most common is to walk my stretch of beach. It has lessons of patience and compassion to teach, and it is one of my favorite teachers. Last night we had a wind warning here in Galveston, and the waves washed high and wild, beyond the fences of the beach houses, eliminating the walkway I use. Tonight, there is a full moon, a clear sky, a brisk breeze, and the beach is stretched out fifty yards from the beach houses, meeting softly breaking waves almost silent in their steady murmur.

These are only two moods of the sea. There are what seem to me at least fifty others. As someone raised inland, I am always startled by their complexity and variance. I love this sea, but I also know that I could study it and study it and still not fully grasp the vast complexity of all these moods, all the stuff it throws up onto the land, sometimes taking it back the next day, sometimes embedding it in the land forever. Learning compassion seems that way to me also. It takes the patience to learn more and more until I begin to be able to feel with another, rather than merely standing on the outside watching and judging. It takes openness to the variance and complexity and an awareness of my limits as a learner. It takes time.

A Story

My best teachers of compassion have been patients I cared for. Early in my career, I worked as a staff nurse at a state psychiatric hospital on a unit for children eight to eighteen years old. These kids were mostly street kids, many with behavior problems directly traced to fragmented or conflict-ridden homes. Relationships with parents were often destructive, and many of the kids had been physically abused. It was easy to feel compassion for the kids, often difficult to feel compassion for the parents.

On weekends, like clockwork, a few of the kids would "run," leaving the hospital without permission. Frequently they would be returned by the police.

Sometimes they had gone home only to be beaten again. This would anger, frustrate, and discourage me. One day, I was walking with one of the boys who was a regular "runner" and had just returned the day before, beaten as usual. I was gingerly discussing his weekend with him. Finally, I sort of blurted out, "Why do you go home, Mike, when you know you're going to be beaten?"

He sensed my feelings, something these kids did easily. "You know, a lot of staff don't seem to understand. You may not like my momma, and you may not like what she does to me, but you know, she's the only momma I got." I have never forgotten this lesson. Mike knew compassion better than I, in his way.

Strengthening Through Compassion

Compassion seems to me a gift given and returned in the learning. If you are willing, the negotiation itself can teach you greater compassion. If you listen closely to others, try to hear what they are saying and also what they are not saying, what they are feeling and what they are trying not to feel, you begin to know and understand the dimensions of their humanness: the fears that blind them, the courage they show despite the odds, the confusions that keep them from their own joy of living. If you come to a negotiation committed to compassion, you actually hear differently. Too often, we enter a negotiation if not to win then at least to hold our own. That distorts our perception. It prohibits compassion.

Compassion can also diffuse a fixation on dominance power and simplistic "win-lose" agendas, both for those who have dominance power to exercise and for those who come to the table without this power. There is no assurance that this will occur, but if you bring compassion to the table, you increase the possibility. Without it, the possibility will probably not emerge. Compassion for yourself also keeps you from engaging in self-destructive behavior or consenting to proposals that could harm you or others.

I have found that there are some situations where it is easier for me to be compassionate than others, and there are some people for whom I feel a spontaneous compassion more readily than for others. While I am glad to have a few places where I can easily enjoy the rich benefits of compassion, I find I sometimes have to be deliberate and focused to manifest compassion. If I am invited to an uneven table, the unevenness itself makes it easier for me to abandon compassion and to miss the opportunities it offers me.

As a nurse, working for years with physicians who did not evoke a spontaneous compassion has been a struggle for me. When I began to realize that this narrowness harmed and inhibited me, I made a commitment to learn and grow beyond it. I was fortunate to work with a physician colleague who was willing to patiently teach me the dimensions of compassion I had neglected in my appraisal of his colleagues. While my concern with systematic injustice toward and exploitation of nurses did not diminish, I did learn some new ways of seeing reality, some new compassions.

I discovered that nurses often keep the problems that offended me going by not being honest with physicians. I discovered that we nurses do for physicians what we would best let them do for themselves, and that sometimes we do this because we want their approval. I discovered that the manipulative behavior that nurses use is as destructive as physician control, and that in this fashion we each victimize the other. I learned that there are no victims if there are no victimizers, and there are no victimizers if there are no victims.

Over time, I acquired a more complex and comprehensive sense of compassion; in the process, I saw many realities more clearly. One of the nice things about compassion is that if you take the time to learn it, you discover it has enormous depth and complexity and thus enlarges your window on reality. This enables you to be more complete, more enriched by life. It looks as if it is a gift to someone else, but it is also a gift to yourself. Compassion thus can strengthen your integrity, increase your ability to go to surer and deeper places, and remove distortions from your truth telling. It also tends to feel good to just about everyone.

St. Elizabeth's Operating Room

Reading and into, being takes form,
takes laughter, takes storm
in its stride,
takes loosely the pride
of a song, we must sing
this thing,
harmonize the impeccable,
the wreckable,
balance the paradox, query,
take on casually the mystery.

Turning backward and salt,
we halt
a present gone deliriously past
in the cast
of dies
that shape our demise.

We'll move on,
gone
with the song caught
tenaciously, sought
murmuring in floors,
competing in corridors
with the rigorous immediate now—
how?

Young man with a broken head, barely broken heart,
takes the stage for a brutally broken part,
and we find reasons for being,

for seeing
to details of speed,
reason to heed
the persons, the place,
take our part in a race
so human, so true,
transforming our is into do.

Life learns a shape
from reverence to rape
we project our designs,
our lines
of living on a public screen,
magnificent, mean;
we grasp glimmerings in the tedium,
the contrast of each new medium.

Plurality of lives
will not apologize
for the joy of incipient whys,
lies
give out dogma, complete
and replete
with a well-closed door:
we shall ever deplore
a today without a tomorrow
to heal both our joy and our sorrow.

We retreat, and we realize
all that we visualize:
work, play, and our private designs,
all in its time soon resigns
to the fact that it's more than it seems,
leading out, past improbable dreams.

—pbk

It takes a consciousness of purpose to develop compassion and to invite it to the uneven table. You may actually want to set a chair for it, to announce its presence, to make it a rule of the process. Introducing the possibility may itself prove useful. If persons at the table are unwilling to honor compassion, you already know a great deal about the negotiation you are about to enter. If persons at the table do not know what compassion is, you already know a great deal about the outcomes. You may want to ask yourself why you are at such a table, and what would keep you there.

Acknowledging Cultural Deterrents

The image of compassion in this country often has a connotation of weakness, passivity, a "womanish" quality, viewing woman as inferior and ill suited to the harsh challenges of life. It is often viewed as a "nicety" that serves as a salve when the warrior comes home from the rugged world of commerce and competition and is eased from "his" burden. This image of compassion is often used to explain it away, to say it is appropriate for the warmth and affection of an intimate relationship but plays no role in the "real" world, which is full of cruelty and viciousness.

I was raised with this worldview, and like many women of my generation, was taught that if I wanted to compete in a "man's world," I would have to forgo compassion. I was told that it would prevent me from being "successful." Thus, the very humanizing qualities that women claimed to bring to the workplace were also systematically discouraged. This has been a difficult challenge for me and for many other women. The message tends to be "OK, so you want to play with the big boys; let's see what you can handle!" This is used to engage in all manner of destructive and hurtful behaviors; it often turns up in my professional life to this day. It has also seduced an amazing number of otherwise very competent but dangerously ambitious women.

Rather than feeling that my compassion is welcomed in these environments, I have often had the sense that since no one else gets to be compassionate, it is not permitted of me either. Clinging to the goal under these conditions can be very challenging. When I do manifest compassion, it often evokes discomfort, discrediting, or retaliation. I describe this in my own head as the "sparring cere-mony." If I tell an academic colleague that I wish to collaborate with "him," the most frequent first response is "OK, honey, let's see what you're made of; let's test your mettle." This is followed by the "cyn-icism ceremony," which tends to communicate "OK, honey, what are you really trying to get from me?" If I survive these charades, the third is usually, "But let's never forget who's in control here, OK!" I can survive these tests, but the effort is at best tedious, and the temptation to strike out or strike back is always there. Because it is repetitious, it is also boring. The best part of this reality is the strengthening of compassion that these experiences provide.

Just because others do not decide to take the risk of compassion, to accept the challenge to humanize the planet in a strengthening way, to have the courage to be compassionate despite the odds, does not mean that I have to follow suit. After fifty-eight years, however, the repetitiousness makes me weary. I have studied long and hard to get access to environments where I have hoped to introduce a more humane model of discourse. I have learned the language and the mores. I often wonder why there is no slight spark of curiosity that would ask, "And what is your model of reality, and how might it enrich me?" The rigid need to cling to obsolete models of reality tests compassion but also demonstrates how sterile the dominant paradigm has become in its imbalance. It saddens me in one way but strengthens my resolve in another.

this gift comes

this gift comes
lumbering in light,
sparking soft nuance
and silent comprehension:

feinting and dodging,
warding off flames
as if truth brandished
a weapon, a knife.

this gift stands
away, far enough from
the heart, safe in shadow,
veiled in self-reflection:
struggling and posing,
testing out ideas like
new clothes, sensing the
nakedness escalating.

this gift fades
at any small request, any
promise made or given, the
slightest whisper of yes:
slick, clean, uncluttered,
untouched, untouchable,
safe in deadly dangers
of elaborate illusion.

this gift shines
despite the fogging farce,
within the swirl of smoke,
through the film and dusting:
shines ablaze, shines sunny,
shines feather soft and light,
shines through all the careful
scripts, the decision to never shine.

this gift leaves
no traces in the sand.

    —pbk

Any worldview that needs that much defending, that comfortably inflicts that much harm, clearly needs a dose of compassion. Realizing this has helped me a great deal. I still am unimpressed with the resilience of my compassion, and fervently wish I could develop it with greater ease and with the positive assistance of others, but I do not doubt the worth of the goal. No one needs compassion as much as someone who thinks it doesn't, can't, or won't exist in their lives. The poverty of spirit implicit in this worldview sometimes seems overwhelming to me.

Learning Humane Discourse from the East

I have said all of this for a reason. Most Westerners struggle with compassion as if someone were telling them to lie down in front of a speeding Mack truck hell bent on driving over them and then to smile beatifically at the driver. I've said what I've said because I know the feeling. It has taken me a long time to learn a more resilient, realistic, and robust conception of compassion. You too might find that learning more about compassion is worth the time.

I have found Eastern literature especially compelling and helpful. One such resource is the I Ching, an ancient Chinese system of divination and book of wisdom. I turned to it first because psychologist Carl Jung had used it to activate his unconscious wisdom, and I wanted to learn about that process. Over the years, I have returned to it repeatedly. It is for me an inexhaustible resource. The most recent version, of the many I own, has a tone more congruent with Western images and has been most useful to me (Walker, 1992). One day, out of curiosity, I decided to record the central principles that recur in this version of the I Ching, which I consider a book of compassion.

The I Ching captures principles as human qualities. This is the list I generated: *balance, modesty, patience, acceptance, humility, moderation, equanimity, tolerance, gentleness, caution, reserve, innocence, generosity, allowing, good, serving, independence, inner truth living, inner strength living, correct behavior, perseverance, attentiveness, adapt-*

ability, detachment, disengagement from evil, receptiveness, openness, reticence, and alertness. After you read this list, you need a huge dose of compassion for yourself so that you don't despair. Then, if you reflect on them for a while, you begin to notice how all of them, combined, would be a superb way to be at any table, anywhere, any-time. It is in this sense that I think compassion has the power to enrich and inform.

Often we are unwilling to believe in the power of principles such as these and feel it is too unsafe at an uneven table to manifest these central principles, to truly be compassionate. Usually we believe we will lose something or be abused or exploited if we do. We read this list with a Western mind, or believe others at the uneven table, incapable of thinking otherwise, will experience our behavior from a Western perspective. The quest for compassion thus asks us to trust that the surer and deeper place, the truth, and personal integrity tempered by compassion can move a negotiation to a bet-ter outcome.

To never test the question is to admit defeat before the race. To bring compassion to the table, to seat compassion, and to keep com-passion there for the whole negotiation asks a great deal, but to do otherwise ensures a great deal less than might have been. With compassion for myself and others as my companion, my clarity of judgment is enhanced. It becomes a bright light I can shine on every dimension of a negotiation. If I am equal to the challenge, if I run that race, I will never be diminished by a negotiation. Look-ing back, those negotiations that have diminished me have always involved a lack of compassion, either for myself or for others. That look in the rearview mirror has been of great value to me.

———————

An Exercise

Facing your own assumptions about compassion at an uneven table can be tough. It helps to know what you really think and feel about something before you rashly invite it to a table, especially one where you might feel vulnerable or at risk. This exercise gives you a chance to check out some of your views on compassion.

You'll need your journal for this. That didn't surprise you, did it? You should be grateful to me. I could have suggested that you go out and find ten people who drive you bananas and try out some compassion on them. Instead, you get to search, in the privacy of your home, for the indicators of your own real sense of this human quality. When you finish the exercise, however, you might have a better sense of what is going on between you and those ten people. You may not be more compassionate, but you may be more honest about compassion in your life.

Remember the list of human qualities from the I Ching? How could you forget, right? Well, write them down in a long column on a page of your journal, with lots of space beside them. Next, make a column titled "I Am" and beside each quality, indicate the strength of the quality you believe you have, using a scale of zero, meaning none, to ten, meaning in full measure. Reflect on this for a while.

Now make a second column headed "Like in Others" and do the same rank order. Compare the two columns. Pretty interesting, isn't it? Make sure you don't cheat with this exercise. The greater your candor, the more you learn. You don't have to submit your journal to anyone, but keep it in a safe place.

Now make a third column, and at the top put the name of someone you really admire, love, or respect. You can actually do this part several times, making as many columns as you like. For now, do one. Compare the outcomes to those in the first two columns.

Finally, make a fourth column, and at the top, put the name of someone who drives you bananas. One of those ten people I mentioned earlier will do. Use the same scale to estimate the person's qualities as you experience them. As is obvious, you can also do this fourth column often.

Comparing the four columns is useful for a variety of reasons, some of which will seem quite private to you as you do so. Now imagine that the three concrete people you ranked—yourself and the other two people—are playing Bridge or Monopoly or discussing politics at a party or possibly trying to determine where to purchase the best produce in your community. Seat yourself at the table and picture the discourse for a while. Was compassion invited or not? If not, invite compassion. Was it hard to find a seat for compassion? Did you know what compassion would do if invited to the table? How could you tell that compassion was really there? What happens with compassion there? Did you like it or not? Why or why not?

This exercise occurred only in your head, on paper, and in your imagination. What would happen if it occurred in real life? What do you think of that question? How do you feel about your answer?

———————————

21

Way of Being Number Five
Draw a Line in the Sand Without Cruelty

If you struggled your way through the last way of being, this one might bring you some comfort. It also might be timely to recall that none of these ways of being are considered independent or uninfluenced by any other: they are a field of action, a gestalt, and to introduce one without the others leads to the imbalance I have been so energetically distancing myself from throughout this book.

Claiming and Creating

When I started studying conflict resolution, I was in the midst of the adventure of a Kellogg Leadership Fellowship and joined several other "fellows" in pursuing this area of interest. We had a variety of learning experiences, many of them from the sagest leaders in the field. It was an exhilarating and expansive process for me. One insight among all others, however, had a great impact on me. It has proven to be the most valuable lesson I've learned.

In discussing conflict resolution, it helps to differentiate between those who come to a negotiation to "claim" that they must prevail and those who come to a negotiation to "create" a solution to the conflict. This is probably a somewhat artificial distinction, since I have never sensed myself or others as fully creative, without some sludge of "claiming" stuck in their system. Still, one or the other intent often prevails. This isn't the insight—it's just the prologue.

The insight involves outcomes between such parties. It is quite simple: if two claimers negotiate, the outcome will be the most limited and unimaginative one possible. Each will get something, but it will be minuscule. If a claimer and a creator negotiate, the claimer will always win. (I know, this is awful news; I'll return to it in a moment.) If two creators negotiate, the outcome can exceed the predicted possibilities. (This is the good news that helps temper that bad news about claimers!) It is also why conflict resolution makes such good sense, why it is a preferred option.

When I learned the second insight, about claimers always winning when seated with a creator, I sputtered myself into a frenzy, demanding a recount on the statistical analyses with the game theory research that had demonstrated clearly: claimers always win in a negotiation between claimers and creators. It offended my sense of justice, my hopes, and my fantasies. Since I usually come to negotiations as a creator, the theories were telling me that I was always going to lose if there was a claimer at the table. Sounds familiar, doesn't it!

The teacher, who as I remember it, was Howard Raiffa (1982), patiently explained that indeed claimers always win but that this need not inhibit me. I was suspicious. "What do I do, then, when I realize I'm trying to create and the other person is claiming?" I had grown desperate by now.

"You say, 'Excuse me, I came to this negotiation in the hope that we could together create some resolution to our conflict acceptable to both of us. It is my impression that you are here exclusively to lay claim to the outcome you want. I need to know if my impression is accurate or not. Can you tell me?'" There tend to be two major possibilities here: yes or no. Actually, in my experience, the yes and the no aren't always quite that clear, but the overriding answer tends to be discernible—if not immediately, at least over time.

If the answer is, "No, I too came here primarily to create," you can continue with the negotiation in the hope that two creators can generate outcomes that exceed the predicted possibilities. This is pretty exciting, because it means that the outcome is only limited by our collective imagination and commitment.

If the answer is, "Yes, it's true, I'm here primarily to lay claim to my preferred outcomes," you have another set of choices. You can then join in the claiming agenda and each take turns in a desperate attempt to win. In the end, the outcome will be limited for both of you. This is the most common model, and it entails long-term harms that sometimes do not resolve themselves before death visits one of the parties. It is an option, however, especially if you like sparring for its own sake or feel you have no choice. Many court cases look this way to me.

If the answer is, "Yes, it's true, I'm here primarily to lay claim to my preferred outcomes," you can take an alternate route. You can say, "Well, I choose to only be here if I can create. Since you choose to claim, I already know the outcome. You will win. Therefore, there is no sense in my staying at this table. I am leaving." Then you leave the table.

This was revolutionary thinking for me. We who have been schooled into beliefs about our own vulnerabilities in negotiations, who believe we are always at uneven tables, didn't have that one on our list of options. If you accept your victim status, you tend to believe that you have to stay at the table or horrors will visit you and your loved ones. In some rare cases, this is actually true. And even then, it is a choice. In many cases, however, it is not. When it is not, simply leaving is an option.

leaving

> *scrubbing down everything helps*
> *rearranging sweaters and spoons,*
> *scissors and salt, the pillowcases.*
> *digging up everything helps:*
> *hoeing, spading, raking, and bagging*
> *last year's harvest and weeds.*
> *leaving helps.*

> *—pbk*

Because I liked to think of myself as creative, I thought I should stay at the table in perpetuity, until I grew hoary and old and cranky. I would just keep saying, "I'm here to create!" and hope for the best. I didn't quite realize how perseverating this was at the time. In retrospect, I realize that I have overstayed my welcome numerous times because I failed to put "leave the table" on my list of options.

Now, with it added, I realize I had a whole new array of decisions and challenges. I needed to know what would make me leave the table. I needed to know my "bottom line." That is how I discovered the importance of drawing a line in the sand without cruelty. I learned I needed to draw the line. I have put it in the sand, because I have learned over time that if I can draw others into a more positive agenda, I can move the line. Having it in the sand helps. If another person manifests compassion, or goes to a surer and deeper place, or becomes a truth teller, or explains components of personal integrity that clarify my understanding, I can adjust the line.

I would like to think that the phrase "without cruelty" would be self-explanatory, but just in case, I will comment. The need to draw a line in the sand can be discouraging. You might like to think that others at the table know you have such a line. It gets wearisome trying to deal with people who need to be told what to you is obvious. It is easy to become cruel in doing this. That is why I mentioned it.

Noticing Cooptation Early

Negotiating at an uneven table is always a challenge. If you are the disadvantaged person, you know you are not privileged and that since the table was set without acknowledging this, you are entering a process with a set of expectations. The assumption is that you are present to help resolve a conflict. Negotiators, and sometimes others at the table—both those advantaged and those disadvantaged—often ask that each person pledge at the outset to avoid creating further conflict. They can thus, even inadvertently, draw you into being creative when others, by reason of unacknowledged privilege, will be actively claiming.

During such a process, solutions tend to be introduced that sustain societally structured inequity. That which was unjust at the outset is continued by the generation of solutions that assume sustaining the injustice. I am not saying that in such a case people are being mean, nasty, and ugly. They may, and often do, simply create out of their own reality, not realizing the limits of that reality. It may never occur to them that an alternate reality exists, or that theirs would not prevail. If they are accustomed to exercising dominance control, they often think it is the natural order of things and can't imagine some other "unnatural" approach. Thus, no matter how creative the solutions appear, they will simply involve shuffling the same set of building blocks. Introducing Tinkertoys would merely confound the process and make no sense to them.

So far, I'm sure the process looks familiar to you if you've sat at uneven tables fairly often. This way of being is designed to interrupt this stagnant "business-as-usual" process, and so it takes some initiative. After struggling through compassion, this might cheer you up at least temporarily. The initiative aims to create, however.

If you are confronted with situations like this, you need to do your homework and know exactly what you will and will not accept with respect to perpetuating injustice. You need to know your line in the sand, and you can only know that if you come prepared for the possibility of an invitation to the perpetuation of an injustice that you choose to reject. If you have some degree of knowledge about a situation, and can acquire additional knowledge, you can usually do this homework. It takes time and energy, but no more than that required to repress rage and fury when the invitation is proffered as if you would foolishly accept it.

A Story

Early in my career, I worked as a surgical nurse and discovered the meaning of a line in the sand. I once was assigned to be the "scrub" nurse for a physician who was chief of surgery. He was a competent, kind, and gracious man, and I welcomed working with him. I had only been working in this department for a few weeks and wanted very much to show my skill and competence. The procedure itself was relatively uncomplicated and went smoothly.

One of the tasks of the scrub nurse was to count the number of pieces of gauze—called sponges—both before and after the procedure. This was done with a second nurse, who validated the count. The purpose was to make sure that no sponges were inadvertently left inside a person during a procedure. As the surgeon begins to prepare to suture closed an incision, the count is done.

I, and the nurse working with me, began our count. We were one sponge short. I told the physician. He said I had probably miscounted. We recounted two more times, while he proceeded to continue to suture. He noted that I was relatively new and suggested that I had simply miscounted or misplaced a sponge. I assured him I had not. He kept suturing.

I stood there flustered, wondering what I was going to do. I knew that my sponge count was correct. I also knew that he was convinced that I was in error and he was not. Finally, I said to him firmly, "You need to know that I will not sign the surgical procedure sheet validating that the sponge count was correct." He was visibly irritated and turned to me and said, "Are you serious?" I firmly but nervously answered yes.

He rapidly became angrier and asked the supervisor to call for an x-ray. All the sponges had a radiopaque strip in them so that they would show up on an x-ray. The portable x-ray machine was brought up, the picture taken, and the machine parked in the room while the technician ran downstairs to develop the film. On his return, the x-ray was posted on a light frame in the surgical suite. The radiopaque strip of one small sponge stared at all of us. It had already been sutured in.

The sutures were removed, the sponge located and removed, and the case was completed. I shook through most of the rest of the very silent and tense process and felt the disapproval and frustration filling the room. It was an early life lesson for me. Despite the reaction to my line in the sand, I at least had the knowledge that the patient did not leave surgery with a sponge in her abdomen and a potentially worsened condition from this effort to help her with surgery. The surgeon said nothing more to me and left the room. We never spoke after that. I learned the impact of a line in the sand. I also learned the necessity.

The events that followed taught me more. Privately, this physician advised the operating room supervisor that he would no longer be doing any surgery, that this event had convinced him that he should no longer be doing operations. I was deeply saddened by this, since he was a very good surgeon and a very good person.

His decision taught me the price of dominance control, the cost we all pay when persons believe that they must control all outcomes, that they may never make a mistake, that others cannot be trusted to keep them from error, and that failures in these efforts require self-punitive responses. Had he not believed that dominance control was the only approach to negotiations available to him, he might have chosen to operate with the assumption that I too could make a contribution that could benefit not only his patient, but also him.

Communicating Your Line in the Sand

Once you have clearly identified your line in the sand, you need to take the responsibility to clearly communicate it to others at the table. You need to do this despite the fact that this may temporarily increase the level of conflict. If it does, you need to activate all the other ways of being to work with the conflict until you can determine the actual response to your line in the sand. If others react to your line negatively, it is easy to slide into cruelty. Standing your ground during this phase is critical.

As you observe the responses to your line in the sand, you can begin to ascertain the degree to which the table was set with the assumption that you would "go along." You can determine if others plan to "go along" and if anyone else at the table has a line in the sand. You can begin to grasp the depth of attachment to an injustice and the resilience with which others intend to protect this injustice. If people become cruel, you can learn how far others will go to protect their claims. This information is necessary to determine if you should stay or leave, but it also tells you the nature of the investments at the table in keeping the table uneven. If you are

not the negotiator, it is especially important to determine the negotiator's stance on your line in the sand.

As you can see, I am recommending that you do this as early as
possible in the negotiation. I once thought waiting a tasteful period
of time was in order, getting to know folks by sipping punch and
nibbling cookies. What I learned from doing this was that if my line
in the sand is introduced well into negotiation and people had fervently hoped I would "go along," my sudden clarity can make others feel tricked or betrayed. Having others do this to me has had the
same impact. This has convinced me that it is wiser, albeit more difficult, to draw this line early and clearly.

In a culture such as ours, where competitiveness is so pervasive
as to be viewed as inevitable, it is important to determine the best
way to draw a line in the sand. It is easy to destroy this way of being
and draw your line in a manner that others experience as a challenge to a contest or an act of assault and battery. But you do not
have to bludgeon others with your line in the sand; you can draw it
with gentleness and grace. It may require repetition, but your
approach can be civil and compassionate, yet clear. Clarity and confidence are more valuable than force and aggression for this gesture.

Still, the culture will often prevail. If you don't turn the line
in the sand into a contest, some folks will believe that maybe you
didn't really mean it, or maybe it is actually just nicety, or perhaps
you can be seduced, cajoled, or coerced into thinking differently.
They will try. For such persons, a more direct approach may eventually be called for. You do not have to start there, though you
should be prepared to go to that degree of forcefulness if necessary.

At an uneven table, more submissiveness and compliance will
often be expected of you because many people think that this is simply the natural order of things. You have to remind yourself that it
isn't. Sometimes you will be the only person at the table who knows
this. You may also be the only person drawing a line. The most common problem I have experienced with this is the "quick agenda."
Someone conducts a meeting with the outcomes predetermined by

others and calls me in to bless it with a formal dance. I am called in because I am one of the people who are supposed to have a voice in the decision. This is called democracy in some persons' lexicons.

When I challenge the decision—when I question the injustice or impropriety the decision reflects—I need to be prepared to say why I am slowing down the "quick agenda." I can easily be labeled an obstructionist, especially if I am the only one at the table raising certain issues. I need to be ready for active silencing. I have found I need to be prepared to clearly demonstrate that my submissiveness and compliance with the choices of another are not, in my mind, the natural order of things and that I do not choose to give the appearance of consenting to that belief, no matter how compelling it is for others. I also have to be prepared to accept the consequences of my statements. I have learned over the years that if you draw a line in the sand clearly, the consequences sometimes can be cruel and destructive in nature.

Feeling Anxious in the Process

Many times, I just don't like to do the things I have described. I find myself feeling disadvantaged to start with. I then feel like I'm taking on the role of "problem participant" who refused to "go along" when everyone else agreed that the solution was perfect, or at least good, or the best we could do. I usually feel threatened and anxious, because I already know that some people at the table perceive me as inferior, and my perceived recalcitrance will simply evoke even more negative appraisals. Like everyone else on the planet, I would like to be admired, appreciated, and given nurturance and warmth and affection. Sometimes I just get scared.

This requires vanity homework for me. It also requires that I keep myself grounded in my surer and deeper place, that I recall my commitment to being a truth teller, that I honor my personal integrity, even at a high cost, and that I show compassion toward myself and others. I have learned over time that it is important to me to have a strong and caring support network of people who value me for who I am. I need to know that they exist, that they know and love me, and that I can count on them. This sustains me when I find myself facing people who do not want to hug and embrace me for drawing my line in the sand. Though I can commit to trying to avoid cruelty, I cannot assume others have made that commitment, and I cannot count on that to keep my clarity about my line in the sand intact.

Often the line in the sand requires that facts usually "politely" ignored be disclosed. Everyone at the table knows them, but there is a "gentleman's agreement" to deny, silence, or protect these facts. I have to first make sure that I have not accepted this "gentleman's agreement," no matter how wonderfully it is offered to me. If I cannot go to a table on those terms, it is not a table I choose to be at. If, at the table, I reveal the silenced facts, others may not welcome the gesture. Yet if I fail to reveal these facts, I become party to self-exploitation, to harms to others, and to the refusal to take the risk of truth telling. It is a difficult, sometimes painful choice, but it is the one that is before me.

A Story

I was once invited by a faculty colleague to write a chapter for a book. He invited me with a very flattering letter and noted both in the letter and in his book proposal that the most competent scholars on the topic at our university would be presenting their ideas on the theme. He had attached a list of twenty-five of our colleagues. I was the only woman.

I realized immediately that there were several other women on campus who could make very substantive contributions to this book. I knew some of them were actually more knowledgeable than some of the men listed as potential authors. I believed most members of our academic community would concur in my judgment. Thus, he was inviting me to receive the honor of being the only woman author while ignoring my women colleagues.

I called him to discuss it with him. He agreed that many of the women I mentioned were indeed competent but emphasized he didn't want to include them. I noted that his proposal said he had included the most competent scholars on our campus; excluding these women made this statement untrue. He wavered, then said that perhaps I had a point but he had asked me and I was surely the most competent of the lot.

I could hear the tiny voice of personal vanity trying to seduce me. It wasn't worth the price of my integrity, however, or of being a public participant in a denial of the competence of my women colleagues. I told him that I would not write the chapter under these conditions. He accepted my refusal. He never did publish the book consisting exclusively of contributions by male authors described as the most competent scholars on the topic at our university.

Facing Ambiguity

It is not always clear which path to take when one tries to find a line in the sand. The choice often involves a disadvantage no matter which path is chosen, and one must be prepared for this ambiguity. I have found that I must depend on my own inner sense of the best solution to the situation and be prepared to take a stand no other person might elect to take. Since I elected not to be in my colleague's set of authors, no women were represented. Yet, had I consented, I would have publicly diminished many competent women. The choices are often difficult.

There is a danger in drawing this line that one merely engages in a variant of self-righteousness. The potential for self-deception can be great. To draw a line in the sand may merely be grandstanding or could be an effort to impress others, to be rebellious, or to seek the admiration of the downtrodden. These threats to authenticity have to be acknowledged and explored. Often this is a more challenging task than actually drawing the line in the sand. It has certainly required more demanding self-honesty of me than merely drawing the line does. Hence, it is important to remember that homework is critical. It is also important to remember that all the various ways of being interact. By way of example, compassion always alters how I draw a line in the sand, making my choice to avoid cruelty apparent. Yet, without my line in the sand, my personal integrity is always at risk.

Drawing a line in the sand almost always makes me long for the good old days when manipulation was still being marketed to me as the model of choice. Over the years, I have learned to appreciate manipulation's popularity. There are days when it does look attractive, when I would like just once to go to an uneven table without having to enact this particular line-drawing ceremony. The temptation to be cruel, harsh, mean-spirited, vengeful, spiteful, and attacking is always there, because being dealt with as if one were defective becomes tiresome. It has taken me some time to clarify why all those cruelties are not part of the creative process.

If I choose to become cruel, I merely harm others and may make further harms to others possible through retaliation and greater exploitation. Just as exploiting others harms the exploiter, so also does cruelty diminish and harm me, make me less of who I might have become, and keeps me from the fullness of my own potential. It may offer a temporary satisfaction, but in the end it diminishes me. While this may be hard to remember when others strike out, it is still true, and I have learned over time to trust the truth, even when I am less than effective at manifesting it.

What the claim-create research taught me is that I always have the option of leaving the table. If my line is unacceptable, I can choose to not be part of the negotiation. It has taken me many years to understand that because I come to the table with so much less, I have so much less to lose, and in that sense, have greater freedom. I once thought that it was imperative that I stay at a table, that I was there to represent women or nursing or patients who desperately needed health care. It took me a long time to realize that if my presence deterred the outcomes I embraced, it was better that I not be there. Either way, the injustice would continue. If I stayed at the table, I risked becoming a party to it. Better leaving than cooptation. This has been a hard lesson for me to learn.

Finding the Positive Outcomes

Learning to draw a line in the sand has also had some unpredicted positive outcomes, however, and these capture my energy and attention with more hope. Once people know where I am at, they are often better able to assess their own choices. I have found that some people have drawn the same line but have been too fearful to say so. They become supportive and helpful. Sometimes the person exercising dominance power shares this line but does not feel free to say so. My expressing it can assist in making it a prevailing norm. Sometimes, together, we at the table can create the conditions for justice because we collectively choose to move beyond the assumptions of inequity.

This way of being has taught me that often awareness only emerges if someone, somewhere is willing to draw a line in the sand. Once it is drawn, the conflict and the negotiation enjoy a higher level of clarity. People make better choices and find themselves willing to honor a boundary that better reflects what they know as their personal best. The temporary discomfort of drawing a line in the sand then seems a small price to pay for the creative potential that unfolds. This has happened to me often enough now that I am learning to trust and respect it. It does not make it any easier for me to draw a line in the sand without cruelty, but it does make the struggle for the courage and self-honesty to do so worth the effort.

As may be apparent, the need to draw a line in the sand at an uneven table evokes a degree of reflectiveness that may not be spontaneous. These choices, which I experience as moral dilemmas, require careful consideration. Some crass choices are obvious, but more often the lines one needs to draw at an uneven table are subtle and complex. There are trade-offs, gains and losses to be assessed and accepted. When another person chooses to accept my line in the sand and honors it, that can be very gratifying. When my line in the sand is rejected, I need to be prepared to take the "losses," whatever they may be. My line, and the "losses" I may experience by drawing my line, can have substantial consequences, and I need to accept that possibility before I go to an uneven table. For me, it has become the only way I can stay there, however.

——————

An Exercise

This one is a retrospective. They're easier, in one way, since you don't actually have to go out there and do something as soon as you face a new conflict. They're harder in another way, since they ask you to scrutinize something in the past, something you can't alter. They may unveil new options for the future, however.

I'd like you to go back mentally over conflicts and negotiations you've had in the past. Think of one that was settled but left you feeling unsettled. Perhaps you agreed to something but you're not sure you really feel good about what you agreed to, and it still bothers you. Recall that conflict and that outcome. Write them down. Try to do this in some detail, giving the specifics of the conflict, the negotiated agreement, and the final outcome. Be concrete.

Now write down exactly what left you feeling unsettled. It might be something like, "I thought John got the short end of the stick," or "I thought there were other solutions that we never explored." Try to be very specific. Then expand on this idea. How did you feel about this outcome? What did you say at the time? What did you do at the time? When did you notice that you were feeling unsettled about the outcome? Then? Later? Did you do anything about this? Did it have an effect on your relationships with the people in the conflict? What effect?

Try to write down as much of this as you can, sort of like telling a story or writing a novel. You need not publish this, but the narrative detail will help. Your unsettled feeling should be pretty clear by now. Study it for a while and try to describe it as a "line in the sand." What might you have stated at the outset of the negotiation that would have prohibited this outcome? Examples might be, "I think no one of us should unduly bear the burden in our solution," or "I think we need to take the time to identify all the potential solutions here; I'm not willing to settle on a solution until I feel that we have exhausted our options."

This is a retrospective on the subject of lines in the sand. Often we fail to draw these lines. By reviewing a past event, we may become more conscious of the need to draw such lines, and to begin to imagine how we might state them and what benefit they might bring to all parties to a conflict. If an outcome unsettles you, at some level it probably unsettled everyone. Even the person who seemed to "prevail" is at some level diminished if the participants failed to draw an important line in the sand.

This review of a past event may give you new insights into future options. Whenever a negotiated agreement disturbs you, this exercise may be useful to repeat. In time, you will have identified most of your "lines in the sand." In time, you may even be able to draw them clearly, early, without cruelty.

———————

22

Way of Being Number Six
Expand and Explicate the Context

This way of being moves us toward further enlarging the process we become a part of when we approach an uneven table. If we come to the table as someone worried or preoccupied about its unevenness, we may be so focused on our fears and apprehensions that we will find ourselves constricting and narrowing our field of vision. We will become as small in our minds as those who view us as diminished think we actually are. Thus, coming to an uneven table with a goal of enlarging the process can itself serve to liberate and enliven us, and increase our creative capacities.

Enlarging Reality

If a table has been set that indicates either an intentional or an unintentional acceptance of unevenness, those who have set the table have succeeded in denying some important dimension of reality. Some source of variance was not included in the assessment of evenness. Inequities have gone unacknowledged for some reason. It is not difficult to ascertain this fact if one chooses to focus on it and conduct one's own appraisal.

One way to attend to this systematic bias is to bring all possible sources of variance to the table. If there are no representatives of these diverse sources of variance, one way of being at the table is to identify these unattended to dimensions. These can be clearly stated, and help to expand the context to include systematic inequity factors. If you take the time to evaluate an uneven table, you can usually find what is missing—what dimensions of the conflict are being treated as if they simply did not exist.

A Story

I was once asked to participate in a major university initiative to enhance university-community relationships. The university hoped to become a better neighbor to the surrounding community and developed a major program to address this goal. The goal was to initiate several projects that would enhance the community and thus please the university's neighbors.

At the first meeting, the planners made it clear that substantial changes would be made in the community, some requiring people to relocate, some changing the nature of the neighborhood. There were no references to community input in any of the plans. Rather, the intent was to invite those at the meeting to sell the idea to the people in the community. It was assumed that those of us who were members of the university community would be willing to go to our neighbors with whom we were already engaged in various efforts, and sell this new plan.

While the operative concept was one of partnership, clearly the planners intended to control the initiative and to manipulate or demand community consent and involvement on terms already determined without any community voice. The community was fragmented. Many people who lived in the community were indigent and politically powerless. There was clearly no intention of involving the community in the planning. Rather, the intent was to control the community, to tell it what was best for it, to tell our neighbors that we knew better what was good for them than they themselves did.

I knew this message well, having spent so much of my career having others tell me how visionary and clear they were about what was best for me, and often ordering me to comply. I realized that we were not interested in a partnership with the community but wished only to exercise dominant power to meet our own self-interest. To make matters worse, those of us who had actually gone through the process of listening to community representatives were now being asked to turn on these fidelities, and to manipulate the people who had learned to trust us.

It was clear to me that the dishonesty imbedded in this process was something I was not willing to participate in. Yet I had to acknowledge the invitation and explain my viewpoint. To introduce the presence of systematic inequity, I raised the question of how our effort might be perceived as a partnership. I also suggested that we might hold open forums in the community to provide an opportunity for people who lived in the neighborhood to voice their concerns, preferences, and desires. I noted that we could seek community input through a door-to-door survey. Gradually, these ideas became part of the initiative.

While they did not give the community control of the process, these measures did increase the voice of the community. They also made it possible for me to participate in this troublesome process not as an impediment but as someone who could make a difference. Had I absented myself, these further dimensions might never have been acknowledged or explored. Had I failed to expand the context and then explicate ways of responding to it, I might have merely been coopted. While the outcomes did not meet my personal hopes for an honest and constructive partnership, they did increase the amount of good coming from the process.

In this planning process, had no one raised these issues, the plans would have proceeded without any honest appraisal of the things that were important to the people in the neighborhood. This systematic exclusion of the neighbors, while seeming to act on their behalf, is a useful example of a narrow context. It just seemed easier to get the job done if one did not have to bother talking to the neighbors while fixing up their neighborhood. The expanded context was not necessarily welcome.

You have to be prepared to say "unwelcome" things when you try to expand the context. It has usually been kept confined for a reason, and the effort to expand it will unveil that reason. Often people place boundaries on a conflict because they hope that in this way they will be able to create a simpler or more controlled solution. Often the assumption of dominance power is the only rationale. When you interrupt this assumption, you have to be prepared to absorb the shock waves of others' disrupted denial or petulant guilt. This can be pretty unappealing sometimes. It may, however, be the only way to preserve truth and integrity. Sometimes it even becomes your line in the sand.

Expanding as Disturbing

Some people get disabled when the context is expanded. They have become attached to a worldview with predictable boundaries, and they are reluctant to see the boundaries shift. They intuitively may realize that the implications of this expansion can be substantive. They may experience these implications as threats and be unable to imagine that they might also be opportunities. They may have become accustomed to silent people staying silent, and the new voices may disturb or confuse them. Thus, they may require more concentrated efforts at compassion or require several repetitions of a line in the sand.

Context factors can be powerful. Clearly revealing these factors may unveil denied or ignored aspects of a conflict. Whole new images and pictures may emerge. One way of viewing this is as a source of enrichment: more variables to serve as part of a creative solution, more people to implement the solution. Another way of viewing this is as a source of further conflict. When you introduce context expanding variables, you need to be prepared for those who do not welcome them. Such persons usually are dealing with the threat dimension of the expansion. You also need to be prepared to work actively with those who know that such context factors can be an opportunity for creativity.

A Story

In the 1970s, most campuses in this country evolved through a process of organized efforts by faculty women to enhance the status of women on campus. Like many other women during that era, I was actively involved in this effort. Women faculty formed organizations designed to bring women together for mutual support and to collectively pursue a political agenda of increasing the power and status of women. We found ways to get women on committees, created faculty mentoring systems, supported one another in introducing women's studies courses and programs, and worked to get women into key leadership positions.

These efforts paid off. In time, many more women were tenured, increased numbers held key administrative and committee positions, and women became a more active and credible voice on campus. In time, some women noted that we were not really supporting all women on campus— only faculty women. On my campus, we proposed to expand the boundaries of our organization to include women in a variety of roles other than faculty. The process was instructive.

Over the years, we had all paid a good deal of lip service to the importance of supporting women. We had said we meant all women, despite the fact that only faculty women were involved. We had done much to improve the well-being of faculty women on the campus. Yet when we proposed to expand our context, many faculty women actively resisted. They noted that our problems as faculty were not the same as those of other women, that these other women did not have access to as many options for power and control as faculty, that we had too little in common. The discussion was intense.

The boundaries were expanded. Many of those who had supported the organization slowly reduced their investment, began to skip meetings, and failed to endorse initiatives. Slowly they abandoned the organization. When the context was expanded, the prevailing commitment to sustaining a hierarchy of relationships among women was unveiled. Some faculty women were willing to invest in efforts to help faculty who were women but were unwilling to invest in efforts benefiting secretaries or student advisers or registrars who were women. Thus, it became clear that these women did not really support women, but only those women they perceived as in relatively powerful positions. They had embraced the dominant paradigm of the campus and perpetuated it at the expense of other women.

I have spent the last eight years of my career in an academic health science center, where I revisit these issues in new costumes. Communities of academic physicians, increasingly inclusive of women, are now facing these same challenges, and it has startled me to find recurrent patterns. The women physicians are interested in equity for women in health science centers, but often elect to exclude nurses from this dialogue, or if nurses are included, to covertly assume that hierarchic patterns of relating will persist. They seem reluctant or unable to see that the very gender disparities they experience at the personal level are ones they are electing to perpetuate at the group level, that is, in their relationships with nurses.

Watching my own daughter physician and her peers interact with nurses gives me hope that future generations may find more constructive pathways to walk, however. Perhaps incorporating younger generations that were raised with a more refined sense of gender equity is itself an emergent option for context expansion. I am learning the same kind of hope in the future watching the career patterns of my younger daughter who manages a large retail store. Perhaps the voices of the next generation are always voices of context expansion.

Discovering Boundaries

Perhaps nothing does more to clarify the actual nature of a conflict than expanding the context. It invariably introduces discomforting sources of variance that unveil unstated assumptions. For that reason, it is critical to become aware of people who want to deal with conflicts in a bounded, reductionistic fashion. They usually argue for a form of isolationism but present it as a commitment to discriminating thought: no need to confuse the issue of racism by acknowledging the silent Hmong community, or to confuse the issue of air pollution from auto emissions by noting the committee is chaired by the president of a polluting factory.

This error to eliminate systematic sources of bias must be dealt with in a somewhat persistent fashion, since the silent voice will repeatedly be silenced. It helps to ask people to explain to you why these contextual factors are not germane, why they keep being ignored. It helps here to be clever and quick on your feet, since the silencing is often subtle and swift. Learning to ask good questions is a central skill in expanding the context.

Omissions

Because many who exercise dominant power focus heavily on action as the arena of moral judgment, they are less skilled at realizing that errors of omission are as serious, and sometimes more serious, than errors of action or commission. To have failed to do the right thing is as problematic as to have done the wrong thing. This insight may have to be introduced repeatedly. It does not seem to come easily to people in our culture, who assure themselves of guiltlessness by proclaiming "I did nothing wrong." It is equally critical to determine if one has failed "to do something right."

In my experience, expanding the context requires persistence. It can rarely be done once and for all. This is not necessarily because people are slow to learn or resistant to the insight. It is as often simply a case of lack of consciousness. Habituation to the denial of certain realities is often so deeply imprinted that shifting someone's attention requires repetition and practice. People often need to be reminded. This requires skill, or one quickly becomes perceived merely as a nag and a naysayer. Explicating context can be a reminder, noting now this dimension, now that one, until the entire picture starts to come into focus. Repetition seems needed.

To further interrupt this habituation, it helps sometimes to state that you don't want the negotiation to continue until context factors are clarified: Just how much of reality are we going to acknowledge in this conflict? This becomes something of a line-in-the-sand decision, but it may be necessary if the context factors being ignored are central to the conflict. This also serves to interrupt the tendency to give lip service to efforts at expanding the context without actually doing so.

Perhaps because I have experienced this so often as a dimension of how persons involved in dominant power tend to negotiate with me, I often feel I am being patted on the head in a sort of "Yes, dear, we know what worries you" fashion. While people are kindly, and even say things such as "Phyllis has given us some things to think about here," there is no real intention of expanding or explicating the context.

This can be a trap. People at the table will admire you for your good-faith efforts but may be completely unwilling to change the context or let themselves become aware of the implications of this larger context. They need you to be wrong, albeit as a fine and noble person, so they can get on with their predetermined outcomes. It is critical to be wary of this behavior. It is also important to know yourself well enough to know when your vanity might deflect you from the task of expanding the context. People can make you feel great about what a wonderful context expander you are, admire and applaud you, and never really get serious about expanding the context. If you really know that the context needs to be expanded and explicated, you need to be firm and clear and may sometimes have to refuse to go on unless this happens.

My daughters have been instructive in this process, particularly during their more intense adolescent years. They, like most adolescents, had the uncanny ability to sense all forms of adult hypocrisy during those years and to announce these awarenesses with some fervor. My older daughter observed that if I was troubled by her peers' beer parties, I could act on this by organizing efforts to confront irresponsible drinking behaviors in the parents of her peers. My younger daughter noted that if people really wanted to solve the problem of drug use among teenagers, they might first ask the teens why they used drugs rather than trying to reduce access to the drugs. I have never quite recovered from these bits of advice.

What they realized about me was that I wanted the context to stay narrow, to fit my worldview on how the adolescent world operated and should operate. I wanted to fix the teens and ignore all the context factors created by adults—many of them reflecting frank hypocrisy. They also knew that organizing the parents to get honest with these context factors was not very likely to happen in our community. While I failed to solve the vexing problems of either beer parties or drug use, I at least stayed in a place of truthfulness better, both with my daughters and their friends. This gave me access to work with them to deal with these issues and preserve my integrity in the process.

This lesson was a significant one for me. I knew the rules of parenthood, the popular conceptions of parental control and punishment, and the social support for demanding a standard of conduct from children that we would not honestly embrace for ourselves. I did not like this hypocrisy, but it was clear to me that this was the expectation. Breaking from this illusion was a struggle, but it helped me understand my own propensity for staying entrapped in narrow contexts. It helped me better understand the defensiveness that invariably emerges when the context is expanded in a conflict.

Asking for Clarification

It has taken me some time to realize that I do not need to defend, apologize for, or feel guilty about acknowledging the context factors that I know are germane to a given conflict. All I really need to do is to ask that others clearly demonstrate to me why these factors are not germane. I have learned over time that someone denying reality has more responsibility in a conflict than someone trying to clarify it. If the facts are not germane, I need to be shown how and why. Then, if I am wrong, I need to have the grace to admit my error. The first requirement, however, is to make sure I am wrong.

This can take time, more time than others had hoped to give to the conflict or the negotiation. It is important to know this and to resist the pressure to speed up the process. If I do an ample job of expanding the context, I invariably have a more complete understanding of the conflict and a richer array of variables that might be altered to address it. I also find that if I take the time to do so at the beginning, I won't introduce these later, and waste my time and energy and the time and energy of the other parties to the conflict.

As you add factors and expand the context, you may discover that this frees others to do the same. This can be both encouraging and enriching. Sometimes it helps to do this in a somewhat cere-monial fashion, to elicit from others factors that may not have been noted or focused on adequately. I have found that when I do this, frequently someone will identify a factor that I had denied or ignored and point out my own bias. Once I was complaining to a male colleague that I resented the limits on my freedom that I expe-rienced as a single woman: the places I couldn't safely go, the walks I couldn't safely take, the parking places I couldn't safely choose. He quietly noted that for most men, the same limits existed, since they too did not wish to be harmed, but that no one acknowledged this risk for men.

As factors emerge, the conflict and the context become clearer. As is obvious, silence and reticence do not work in this process. You need to know that you may not get an invitation to expand the context, and you need to know that you cannot assume that others at the table share your view of these context factors. The process of unveiling them, however, can benefit everyone and invariably leads to more comprehensive and realistic solutions to a conflict. Done well, it can serve as the starting point for genuinely creative prob-lem solving.

An Exercise

We're going to branch out a bit now, so be prepared. Up to now, you've been able to conduct all these exercises in the privacy of your own inner dia-logue. This time, we're going to introduce a second party. We will do so ret-rospectively, however, so you don't need to go out and have a nice lively conflict so that you can have something to work with.

Recall a recent conflict with someone you see frequently but feel close to, comfortable with. This may be a partner, a friend, a coworker. Write in your journal a brief description of the conflict as you recall it. Try to select a conflict that was not intensely personal or troublesome, one you would be willing to revisit. Do it with one of the nicest conflicts you've had in a while.

Reflect on your description of this conflict to the person with whom you had it. Do this casually: "Gee, Jane, remember the day we had that tense discussion about my new car," or "You know, Mike, I've been thinking about that conversation we had about the dirty dishes." These are modest openers.

Now, tell the person that you're trying to better understand the way you behave in a conflict. Tell him or her that you want to see if you are missing some factors in such conflicts, if you are leaving out some important insights. Ask the person to tell you about the conflict as he or she experienced it, what was going on for the person, how it looked, felt, and what the person sensed was coming from you. This is a great time to practice being really open, so enjoy it. Let in anything and everything the person tells you, and just listen in a quiet, accepting fashion.

This exercise could make you nervous; I do know that. I did tell you to try an easy conflict. Just revisiting a conflict can sometimes make us want to start it all over again, so work very hard to listen and to hear. Ask questions if this will help you to better understand what he or she is telling you. Get curious. Get involved in the other person's story. Enjoy it. Learn from it. Thank the other person.

Now, return to your journal and list the key points the other person made, the key ideas shared with you. Return to your original description of the conflict. What was missing? The factors the other person shared with you are factors that expand the context. When you asked for more information, you enabled him or her to explicate the expanded context. You have just completed an exercise on the impact of this way of being.

Lest you think this merely a one-time exercise, this model of problem solving can be repeated infinitely. You might just be amazed at how often inviting others to expand their context and explicate it makes it much easier for both of you to ask others to learn of your context factors. Then both parties get to enrich the process and the outcomes. It may seem hard to believe, but it has been my experience that this can even become stimulating and fun.

———————————

23

Way of Being Number Seven

Innovate

I have to admit that this is absolutely my favorite way of being at an uneven table. Some of these ten ways of being are pretty somber and demanding. This one can actually be pretty fun and funny and calls up a lot of my creativity. Thus, you might want to try to relax and enjoy this one as much as possible. There is a playful quality to innovation, a freedom and a release. Innovation liberates and is inherently expansive. Much of the time it feels good. While it can only work in the context of the other ways of being, it's here and yours for the taking.

Clarifying the Rules

One of the first ways of innovating is to seek clarification of the rules at the table. If they don't fit, you can negotiate to change them. Often the rules are set to sustain a focus on dominance power and have built into them all the assumptions, habits of mind and heart, and constraints of the dominant paradigm. Everyone will try to be very linear and logical, the hierarchies will all have to be preserved, patriarchs will emerge on schedule, and the whole process will rigidly force predictive outcomes. Not only is this constraining and unimaginative; it's also pretty boring.

Some examples might be helpful. Sometimes I ask if it is all right with everyone if we come up with ten or twelve great solutions rather than just one. In my experience, people usually laugh, which lightens the atmosphere. They also commit to multiple solutions, which means we can probably craft more interesting and comprehensive solutions. If there is a person overtly identified as the patriarch, I ask him if it is all right with him if someone else gets to be in charge of part of the solution. I usually try to do this with a light touch, with humor. In my experience, unless it is a patriarch hell bent on being one, this is often an attractive alternative, gracefully accepted. This reduces the fixation on dominance power before the process even begins.

These kinds of rule changes are essentially innovations that make it possible to create a process where the other ways of being can become manifest and effective. They serve to interrupt the assumption that the process will be business as usual—a tedious struggle for dominance power. They announce that the traditional ways of being at a table—the manipulations and countermanipulations—need not prevail. If such rule changing is done with a lightness of spirit, it actually changes the context for the process. Then, introducing surer and deeper dimensions, difficult truths, personal integrity, and compassion will seem less dissonant. If done well, this changing of the rules can serve also as a line in the sand.

A Story

One of the challenges facing the health care delivery system in the United States is the rapid change in ethnic demographics in this country. The demographics are of course not the problem but merely point to a set of pressing issues.

Health care in this country has historically been defined, devised, and controlled by people who were European Americans. Much of what has been developed is excellent and shows a wonderful fit with the needs, values, hopes, dreams, and convictions of European Americans. Most of the health care providers find this all quite reasonable, since they too are European Americans. Decades of acknowledging that other ethnic groups existed has been part of this system, but always in a way that asked the patients and their families and communities to adapt to the European American ways of doing things.

As ethnic minorities increase in numbers in this country and as European Americans proportionately decrease in numbers, this ethnic bias becomes more clearly understood as a problem. The health care delivery system needs to change to create responses appropriate to other ethnic groups. The health care providers need to change to provide care appropriate to other ethnic groups. More health care providers are needed who are members of these groups and can help create these changes.

Thus, student recruitment of ethnic minorities into health professions is a pressing need. It is fraught with challenges, however, particularly since many health professions educational programs embrace a covert and unacknowledged systematic racism. These are not easy environments for persons who are objects of that racism to enter. Even more difficult is the challenge to grow, learn, prosper, and lead.

Traditionally, this challenge has been addressed by groups of European American health professionals meeting to strategize, plan, and hope for a solution. When I assumed a leadership position in a school of nursing, I already knew that this approach did not work. The African American leadership in the city where I worked also knew it didn't work and confronted me about it very shortly after I took the job.

I was fortunate in having a good friend and colleague who was a member of that leadership group and served as my adviser. We decided that the best thing we could do was to change the rules. Rather than the school trying to convince realistically skeptical members of her community that we were now a receptive environment, we acknowledged that we indeed were not one but that we were interested in learning how to become one.

We then decided to change the rules even more. We decided that the best way to learn how to become a positive environment for students from the ethnic communities who might consider attending the school was to ask leaders in those communities to assist us. We also realized that in those communities, much as in European American communities, nurses were often passed over as leaders.

We carefully identified the strongest nurse leaders in the African American, Hispanic American, Asian American, and Native American communities. We invited these nurse leaders to serve as an advisory council to our school of nursing to help us learn better how to recruit and retain ethnic minority faculty and students and how to create an environment conducive to growth for all our faculty and students—one where racism could be constructively confronted.

This group met monthly. They were enthused, committed, and creative and sometimes stretched me. They told me what did and did not work, where we were failing and where we were successful. Enrollment of minority students went from eight to fifty-two students in less than four years. We also met with several campus leaders, who began to take note of this "change-in-the-rules" approach to our challenge. Other deans followed suit.

While we clearly did not solve all the problems confronting us, or even most of them, and while resistance can outlast many a good solution, the opportunity to do something really creative and worthwhile, to make a change worth bothering with, came first from changing the rules. Because we changed the rules, we not only created a dialogue that moved us past old conflicts, but everyone benefited. Often changing the rules to a synergistic model with a commitment to openness is enough to precipitate a variety of constructive responses.

Questioning Illusions

Many times, a conflict is sustained simply because popular illusions are sustained and no one has bothered to imagine an alternative. It is thus very helpful, in using this way of being, to practice questioning all sorts of popular illusions. This is more difficult than it sounds. I am perfectly willing to question illusions that I perceive as disenfranchising me or limiting my freedoms. Actually, all illusions do this, especially if they are not conscious. Unfortunately, however, I often am only conscious of this in some cases and totally ignorant and unaware in others. Hence, I may confront popular illusions quite selectively.

Those I hang on to are usually connected with my personal pockets of insecurity and fear. They therefore don't readily respond to being questioned but more often engage in a sort of life-and-death struggle to survive. Hence, this questioning is easy sometimes and very difficult other times. It helps if others join you in the effort. Eventually, someone will disrupt one of your protected illusions and really give you a chance at some freedom. You had better want it a lot, though, or you will merely find yourself starting a new and more virulent conflict.

Innovation is best pursued when illusions can be called illusions. We can then set out to create something a bit more desired and desirable than self-deceptions. Some examples might help here, too. I have found I often have to confront the popular illusion that strong women are inherently dangerous. I have also had others help me confront the illusion that women won't use their strength in dangerous ways. Both illusions are often present at an uneven table, and both are illusions.

Confronting such illusions helps everyone. It increases clarity of thinking and the capacity of all parties to discriminate better. As illusions fall away, the substantive dimensions of a conflict become clearer, and the options for problem-solving effectively emerge, untainted by unacknowledged illusions. While this may be a struggle on occasion, it is ultimately liberating and leads to more reality-based and workable solutions to most conflicts.

Activating Curiosity

Curiosity is a tool of the innovator and should be used liberally and followed when it starts down some sturdy path in the conflict. Curiosity opens you to new ideas. It can encourage you to ask a good question that helps you and everyone else at the table understand the situation better. To ask good questions because you're truly curious about the answers creates a climate of openness that gives everyone access to better information. It also tells other people at the table that you're willing to learn more, to admit that you don't know everything, and to learn from people at the table who know more than you do about something. It can also say that you feel enough compassion for others to want to understand the dilemma from their perspective. Such curiosity can actually become a norm and lead to all manner of unplanned and enriching learning opportunities.

When you're truly curious and open, people tend to tell you more than they might have told you had you never asked. As you listen closely, you find you're better able to understand others, and in this understanding, liberate a good deal more of your own creativity. Relatedness ultimately always serves as a mirror, helping us to understand and express ourselves better. Thus, in the pursuit of curiosity, we find new avenues of discourse, new approaches to our conflict, new ways of imagining a way out of our conflict. We innovate.

There is substantial evidence that the future will probably arrive whether we attend to this fact or not. Most of us most of the time sit around waiting for it, with an occasional effort to stave it off. We look like people watching television, as if the future were something delivered to us over the airwaves rather than something we can choose to create as we wish. This passive stance of letting the future happen to us is an expression of the refusal to own our own lives, to create our own realities. We stagnate when we might innovate. Such inertia is usually harmful. Innovation breaks through this inertia and enables us to create new realities. When our reality is a conflict, choosing to create outcomes that serve the whole can be genuinely innovative.

Since you've been reflecting on the other ways of being for a while now, you might vaguely sense that you too have some rather worthwhile views and hopes and dreams and that these might fit into some larger sense of creating the future. Your contribution is as valuable as anyone's, and in some cases will prove to be more valuable. Passively waiting for the future is often a mental trick of victims. They wait for the delivery so they can call the catalogue company and complain that it is the wrong size or shape or color. If you want a certain kind of future, you need to create it.

If you are accustomed to being at uneven tables, you may assume that those with dominance power will get to create the future. This tends to serve as a self-fulfilling prophecy. Then you get to criticize all the bad people who failed to create a proper future. You may believe you can only create a little piece of the future, but to have done one nice little piece well makes a good deal more sense than whining when the one delivered to you fails to meet your specifications. It is also more fun.

Having Fun

As you might imagine, I've been a little nervous about mentioning to you that conflict resolution at an uneven table can be fun. This may be hard to take in, especially if you're attached to suffering and experiencing pain at the uneven table. This uptight attitude tends to bubble up from fear or blaming, not reality or possibility. Actually, if you feel like you're the disadvantaged person at an uneven table, you have the option of having more fun than anyone else there, especially when the negotiation is about dominance power. All the others are busy protecting their power; you have nothing to protect. You may also become more acutely aware of your own powers, those that heal or confront or hold your ground. These powers are rarely fought over, so they tend to stay intact in such situations.

A good deal of the negotiating about dominance power so popular in our culture is actually pretty funny. When you ponder the truly profound dimensions of human existence, when you reflectively identify that which is most important to you as a human, you rarely come up with dominating others as the top priority. Hence, watching a group of people put that much energy into this goal is actually pretty funny sometimes. It is very innovative to notice this and to laugh as needed or appropriate. It is important to have fun whenever possible, and to acknowledge what is funny whenever possible. As Norman Cousins has taught us, laughter heals.

Understanding Humor

Humor is a complex entity, however, so some guides of action are in order. It is best to avoid stilted jokes; these are merely repetitions and miss the creative moment. It is more innovative to identify dissonances as they present themselves and acknowledge them as they show up in the process. These dissonances are best identified in oneself or in others at the table who are comfortable with themselves. Persons at the table who feel anxious or trapped cannot laugh, especially at themselves. If they had hoped for a quick and easy "win," the fact that you are disrupting this is upsetting, and they quickly become humorless. You need to be prepared for such humorlessness, but you need not be constrained by it.

It is equally important that you not use humor to harm, belittle, or diminish others. Then it is simply a variant on manipulation or cruelty posing as humor. Real humor simply acknowledges the funny nature of much that is human. It is best found in oneself. If others use humor to be cruel, it is important to discriminate. It is also important that you not give cruelty a stage to perform on, with you as hapless audience. Cruelty is actually silly and foolish. Invitations to be harmful can be most effectively dismissed with humor, with the laughter of the innovator who knows there are clearly better ways to resolve conflicts.

Creating New Metaphors

Another path to innovation is creating new metaphors. I actually enjoy this one quite a bit, since I have been working for a long time on trying to find new metaphors to replace all the war metaphors we use. The war ones seem particularly inane to me when I am in the midst of trying to resolve a conflict. Obviously, they subtly sustain the fixation on dominance power and thus are dysfunctional during conflict resolution.

I find it helpful to simply state that I choose not to use war metaphors because I find them inconsistent with the goals at the table. I try to explain that they make me feel like we are actually just engaging in some strange new variant of war called conflict resolution. I am relatively certain that new metaphors create whole new images. I keep working on these so that I have an array available whenever I visit an uneven table.

I think different groups respond positively to different metaphors. Women almost always value the idea of making a quilt as the way we might craft a solution acceptable to all parties, a comprehensive whole that is a synthesis of the parts. Perhaps because so few men have made quilts, this metaphor is less useful to them. For them, the metaphor of harvesting crops we have tended and grown or conducting an orchestra where each instrument plays its part seems to be more acceptable. Learning the metaphors that "work" at a given table is itself a creative activity.

Educating

As is apparent, the goal of much innovation at an uneven table is to educate rather than demand, insist, prevail, or win. People who learn new ideas let these guide their choices. If no new ideas emerge, the old problem-solving behaviors are turned to since no alternatives exist. When you are at an uneven table dealing with inequity, it is important to remember that all inequity is laced with misinformation and ignorance. You can thus use your "air time" to educate those open to the education. The shared knowledge itself tends to disrupt structured inequity and offers new vistas of conflict resolution.

A Story

Academic life offers, among other things, the opportunity to occasionally meet wise people. In the most intensive years of my academic development,

I was fortunate to meet a man who, in many ways, served as the "soul" of the large urban university where I worked. When I could find no other way to solve a problem, I would simply pick up the phone and call him. He always had a solution, and often six or seven. Many faculty considered him a mentor—a role he played with grace and dignity.

He became ill, was admitted to a hospital adjacent to the campus, and was told after an exploratory operation that he would soon die of cancer. News of his plight spread through the campus immediately. It was hard to imagine life without our collective "soul," and the news was deeply disturbing to many people. Some nursing faculty members had been close to him and became actively involved in his care and in working with his family.

Sometimes we were involved in the demanding work of being with someone doing the work of dying, of listening and caring and loving as that process unfolded. Sometimes we helped with simple comfort measures, or assisted the family with plans, discussions, and early grieving. Sometimes we tried to improve the joy of the day with simple gifts or a sign in the school window that he could see from his hospital room.

During this time, many colleagues across the campus began to approach me to ask about him. They were clearly concerned, even grieving. I would encourage them to go visit him, noting that the visits meant a great deal to him, that he would be pleased and would welcome their gratitude for his role in their lives. One after another they demurred. It began to bother me, so I sought further information.

Slowly I began to realize that his illness and death frightened my colleagues, that while they wanted to visit and wish him well, they were too frightened of his death to honestly face him and comfort him. I also began to realize that their absence was hurtful to him. He wondered why they did not come and began to feel the pain of their avoidances.

It is easy to forget as a nurse how deeply this culture denies and avoids death, how we virtually refuse to let it come into our lives without force and even violence. As the culture has steadily deepened its phobic responses to dying, nurses have chosen to stay with the dying more and more consciously. We have always known it is part of the process of living, and that dying well is a gift, too. As the culture has drifted further away, nurses in many ways have become closer to the process of dying.

I had advantages I had not recognized, and I had the support of my colleagues in my efforts.

I had grown accustomed to the absence and avoidance of physicians in the dying process. I realized that often they saw death as a failure and elected to avoid or deny it, arriving only after death to make a pronouncement. I had assumed that my intellectual academic colleagues understood death and would deal with it. I had failed to distinguish between knowing that is of the intellect and knowing that is of the heart and soul.

Here I was participating in the dying of the "soul" of this academic community, and he was as abandoned as the many other persons who had died being avoided by loved ones and friends. I was initially angered by this and needed to reflect for some time before I could solve my dilemma. I decided on an educational way of being.

Since I was in the faculty senate at the time, I asked to be placed on the agenda to speak to the faculty about this issue. I noted that I knew many wanted to bring their good wishes to our friend but were reluctant to go to the hospital, to face the reality of death. I also noted that this man had been so central in so many of our careers that it was simply wrong to fail to be there for him in some fashion. I brought along a large poster and several marking pens and invited anyone who wished to send greetings to write them on the poster.

My faculty colleagues seemed genuinely relieved and eager. Most wrote notes. The poster was taken to the hospital and hung in a place for easy reading, bringing pleasure to both my friend and his struggling family. Many of my colleagues thanked me for this later. I took this occasion to point out how important it is to be there for people when they are dying. They agreed, and while I realized many took only one small step, it was one small step. Without the poster, there would have been none.

This process of attempting to educate is itself relatively instructive. In my efforts to acknowledge the advantage I had as a nurse, I needed to also acknowledge that my colleagues were at an uneven table and that I might be able to help solve their dilemma. Thus, whether I am the advantaged or the disadvantaged person, and usually I am both, I can seek to innovate through education.

It is helpful to remember that those who resist either providing or accepting an education have other agendas, which do not include confronting the ignorance of inequity. For one reason or another, they choose to sustain their ignorance. You need to watch out for such people, who will often indicate that they choose not to learn in subtle ways. When these become apparent, it is helpful to invite them to show you if you are in error and how. If they refuse your invitation, this often indicates that they did understand you, they just didn't like what you had to say because it has unattractive consequences for them.

Education as innovation is particularly useful because it can involve both those advantaged and those disadvantaged, a distinction that becomes harder and harder to make as you study the diverse ways that people feel unevenness at a table. Simply learning more about one another often serves to unveil these assumptions of disparity that are far less rigid than assumed. It also unveils the easy judgments we make about others, about how they could or should conduct themselves since they "have all the power" or "have nothing to lose." Neither statement is ever completely correct.

This dimension of being an educator takes considerable practice. It requires that the course fit the people at the table. It also requires a good deal of self-honesty so that the course is creative and constructive, not aimed at doing harm or belittling those who know less about inequity than you do. It helps to remember that compassion is seated at the table. It also helps to remember that you have drawn a line in the sand. People who persistently refuse to hear you out will often do so by attacking you or discounting what you have to say. This can be disheartening and confusing. Discriminating self-honesty helps. Trusting your own sense of the truth becomes imperative, or you will merely find yourself not only discouraged at the failure to educate, but subtly coopted by permitting the silencing that has occurred.

Becoming a Translator

One of the complex and powerful dimensions of the dominant paradigm is language. The paradigm has a unique language system. Those who embrace this paradigm embrace the language as well. Those who think it is the only paradigm also think it is the only language. People at the table who are disenfranchised have a different language system. Often there are many groups at the table, each with a unique language system. Thus, innovating often requires that you become multilingual.

This is a difficult but rewarding challenge. You have the distinct advantage of knowing that there are multiple language systems, and you are further rewarded when you acknowledge each of them as valid, including that of the dominant paradigm. It is helpful, however, to make it clear that the language system of the dominant paradigm is only one of many. You also need to know which ones you know, and how well you know them. Some you may know little or not at all, and it is important to acknowledge this.

If others use a foreign tongue, request a translation. Often an obtuse language system is used to keep certain people at the table from understanding and participating. To request a translation reveals this ploy and requires that all at the table have an opportunity to learn and understand that language. Sometimes the prevailing language at a table is foreign to everyone but the person who set the table. Beware of this. If it occurs, asking for translations frequently can interrupt this plan. This approach may not be welcome, but it clarifies and gives everyone a chance to learn a new language.

Vanity and insecurity can make it appealing to try to get everyone at the table to understand and speak your language, to understand your reality on your terms. If you are truly at an uneven table, one of the things you can expect is that it is very likely no one at the table will speak your language. It is important to not be surprised when you discover this. It is equally important, however, to use your language once in a while and then provide a translation. It highlights the inequity structured into the negotiation that requires you to sit at an uneven table speaking someone else's language. This keeps the inequity public, in case people are trying to forget about it. Using some of the more interesting and creative dimensions of your language system can help in this effort, making the process more fun. It also serves to educate.

A Story

I once served on a board of directors for a health agency that provided an array of services to underserved communities. The resources for this agency were provided through federal monies awarded to a traditional dominant paradigm institution. Most of the members of the board of directors, however, were members of various ethnic communities. I was the only white woman.

The board members were energetic, committed, and constructive. They knew that what they were doing was important and worked collaboratively to achieve an array of positive outcomes for their communities. Great care was taken to acknowledge "competing" initiatives and avoid favoritism. They were an impressive group of people and gave me the richest experience I have ever had as a member of a board of directors.

As is often the case for white women, my role often reduced itself to serving as a translator between the traditional dominant paradigm institutional representatives and the other members of the board from these various ethnic communities. This was a two-way translation process, although I often felt that each side only perceived one dimension of it. The traditional institutional representatives seemed only to hear me when I translated events into their language. I understood it, indeed spoke it fluently. The members of the board often seemed to only understand me when I spoke their language, which they had painstakingly taught me. The assumptions each "side" made about the other made direct communication difficult.

At one meeting, after I had made several efforts at trying to translate a particular message from the board members and failing, I threw up my hands in spontaneous exasperation and said, "Sometimes it is so frustrating being a white woman!" The members of the board burst out laughing. It broke the tension and we went on. Both the effort at language and the humor saved us from an impasse we might otherwise have been stuck in.

It's hard for me to end a discussion of this way of being, since the possibilities are unlimited, and I want to ramble on and on with stories and examples. It is an inexhaustible source of fun, entertainment, and creativity. It might be best summarized, however, as acknowledging that being creative is almost always wiser than failing to be so. Everything changes; that is the nature of life. Others can "stack" a situation. You can either be disabled by this, or you can innovate. If you fail to do this, it is your failure, not someone else's.

When you're sitting at an uneven table, by its very nature, it includes people who have already told you by setting the uneven table that they like things just the way they are, that they do not want things to change. You need not be startled and amazed by this, nor does it help to become enraged or petulant. It is foolish to expect enthusiasm for change at an uneven table. If people had wanted it, we all would have changed by now. Assume that, and you will have both the ease of mind and soul and the impetus necessary to move you to innovate. You will also have more fun.

An Exercise

This could prove to be both embarrassing and weird, as exercises go, so I am warning you of this fact from the outset. You may discover something about yourself you never fully realized. It will be interesting, though, so you have that to cling to for the time being.

Do you laugh? I hate to be so intrusive, but I'm sort of hoping you can answer with a resounding yes. I'm always a bit startled by the number of people who fight very, very hard to never laugh, even when life gets unbelievably funny. Some cultures do this better than others. Some families do this better than others. Just answering that little question will tell you a great deal.

That's not the exercise, though. The exercise assumes you could remember at least one time in the last twenty years when you chuckled a bit. Eliminating all television, movies, radio, and general entertainment options, go back in time until you can remember an occasion when you laughed. Hopefully, it was only a few minutes ago. But maybe it wasn't. Whenever it was, find it. In your journal, write down a few notes to help you recall the situation, as in, "dinner with Joe and Nancy, recalling childhood stories about fear," or "last night, being teased about my old slippers as family heirlooms." There are no strict rules, except that you actually laughed.

Now that you've struggled to find an example, see how many more you can find. Try to stay in the last five years so you get a sense of recent humor sources. After you have written several down (ten is a nice number), review these and reflect on them for a while. What do they have in common? Was some person a focus of the humor? How often was it you? How often was it someone else? If other people were involved, did they laugh, too? Who didn't laugh? Do you know why they didn't laugh? What actually made you laugh? What made others laugh? Was anyone diminished in the process? Who? Did your laughter break tension or increase it? Why? How? What does humor mean to you, as reflected in these examples? Is this your only option?

You need to get very, very good at this exercise before you can have honest, compassionate, constructive fun at an uneven table.

24

Way of Being Number Eight
Know What You Do and Do Not Know

We all come to conflict and negotiation ignorant in some dimensions, informed in others. This is not a startling insight but a comment on the human condition. This way of being helps you work constructively with that fundamental fact. It first asks you to clearly identify the nature and the boundaries of your knowledge about the issues being addressed at the uneven table. It asks you to do this without defensiveness or sentimentality, without pretense or excuse. It calls forth a discriminating mind, and encourages you to follow the judgments of that discrimination.

If you do this well, you can then evoke a comparable response from others at the table. When you go to an uneven table, especially one where there is a commitment to discounting your knowledge, this process is critical. I usually require myself to clearly identify exactly what I do and do not know about the issues, and state this to myself honestly before I even go to the table. I usually do so imperfectly, but the discipline of the process focuses me and helps me become more discriminating.

It also helps me be less defensive when others at the table begin to indicate to me that I have no knowledge, that my knowledge is too limited, or that my knowledge is irrelevant or incorrect. I can then more comfortably ask others to explicate for me what they do and do not know, and ask of them a comparable level of clarity.

Often persons accustomed to dominant power have little experience in knowing that what they know is limited; they are often left to amble about within those limits as if their knowledge were exhaustive. As a result, they often lack skill at learning about their limits. Thus, soliciting this degree of clarity from them serves to inform them that I know that their knowledge, like mine, has limits. This has also been effective with me when I am not acknowledging or lack awareness of my limits.

Becoming Discriminating

As is obvious, this search for clarity requires that I actively refine my discrimination skills. It has been my experience that in our culture, those who have embraced the dominant paradigm often develop superb discrimination skills. Those who do not often react to this negatively, sensing that the discrimination ignores critical sources of variance, critical context factors. While the scope of the discrimination may be limited or constricted, the skill itself is valuable, however, and I have learned from these fine discriminators. I have benefited from being asked to discriminate with the same clarity and have found I can be more constructive at a table when I am willing to do so.

Often, persons disadvantaged at an uneven table reject these discrimination skills because they experience them within the context of a series of discounting messages, signaling that their reality and their language have been declared invalid. I am convinced that the sense of denied reality is a serious one, but the skills themselves can be invaluable in helping people who are unable to see these realities. By discriminating carefully, speaking in the language of the dominant paradigm, I can often effectively unveil the denial of reality that others embrace. Thus, rather than rejecting discrimination skills, I turn them to a new and constructive use. This has been a powerful and important lesson for me to learn.

half-measure man

half-measure man, boy fist thrust in rage
at a ruthless blazing overhead sun; fragment
searching for a way back to a source, path
to a remembered white light: your sallow eyes
clench tighter than that empty beefy hand.

the knife that cuts a deal, cuts the
heart from every measure; vacuous thought
sulks into power, a tyranny assuring arid
self indulgence, self defeat, alone: not
too hard for a charcoal hardened heart.

outside the uninvaded wall measuring reigns,
naming a winner in the race; you cavort or
gambol, sometimes run. lurking demons or
saints can neither grant a trophy: it is
yours to uncover in that forest, on that path.

i have not broken through your wall, nor found weak
chain links on its gate, but merely loved beyond it
where convergence measures false and true alike,
found nuggets of gold and stones of self-betrayal
on your path: i am not to be blamed for this.

weaving women gather at night to ponder the risks
and gains, discern the possibilities, a process of
dispassionate regard. unmeasured certainties
organic as mulch on the rhubarb are springing
up higher than the moon: this is a dance.

half here, half there, torn like a sterile memo
to a power broker, broken to shreds bit by byte,
you squander time demurring until the night sneaks

in, scavenges you away, rekindles a review of
quality, control: no measures will be taken.

   —pbk

Timing

As this poem makes clear, it is of little value, however, to do this as
if one were trying to assault someone's walls of denial. The insight
will merely bounce off and writhe on the table. It may also evoke
even more rigid denials. One must thus learn to time these inputs
and must proceed with sensitivity, awareness, patience, and caution.
It has actually been my experience that even when my discrimination skills are excellent and my timing impeccable, people can and
do elect to continue to deny my reality and their own. One may
simply have to accept this fact.

This is hard for many people at an uneven table to accept. They
may become frustrated and angry and want to break through the
denial. They prefer the "let's-get-the-bastards!" model of reality testing. I too shared this view at one point but have learned over time
that though it may temporarily make me feel better, since I got to
vent my spleen, I have never seen it either resolve a conflict or
improve the outcomes I am seeking to pursue. It is assuredly not
compassionate and usually does not help others find a surer and
deeper place. It can lead others to a further distortion of their truth
out of defensiveness and creates a line in concrete that merely polar-
izes rather than informs.

Good timing, when it does work, is often creative. Good educators
know that the teachable moment is the best possible moment to draw
a student into a new insight. Being patient enough to find these
moments, to wait for them, asks a great deal sometimes, but it's clearly
more effective than the "let's get-the-bastards" model in trying to solve
a conflict or encourage others to consider surer and deeper places.

To increase my discrimination skills and improve my timing, I
have discovered I need to listen to and learn more actively from

others at the table. I have not come to this awareness either enthusiastically or easily. It has been a great struggle. It has always seemed easier for me to jump in, confront, point out idiotic inconsistencies, and in general ruffle up the process with a little reality. I often fail in my efforts to become the patient learner. Yet, when I do succeed, I find myself better able to know what I do and do not know, and better equipped to engage in genuinely innovative conflict resolution.

Somewhere in the process of learning these ways of being, I discovered that I was really hopelessly inept at this one. To deal with this limitation, I decided I needed to treat the process like a course of study, like a program I had enrolled in because I wanted to learn something. This has helped me sometimes keep quiet when I felt impelled to act or defend, project or blame. It is very hard for me to be patient with people who often seem to know far less about a conflict than I do, yet who tend to talk to me like I have neither comprehension nor reasoning skills. Holding myself to increased refinement of both by learning from others, even those most patronizing, has proven enriching. I really think I'm still not very adept, but I have demonstrated to myself that the lessons are worth the struggle. Often the outcomes are not the ones I had predicted but are noteworthy in their own right.

A Story

I recently attended a national meeting of experts in the ethics of health care. It was the first time I had attended a meeting of this group, though I knew some of its members. I attended hoping to find a meaningful discussion of the profound issues that now face health care providers. The increased technology that controls our care environments has left everyone dazed, discovering that we now have machines that forbid us to die, even when it is our time.

The discussions were surprisingly arid, full of academic rhetoric and theories of how we might all make sound decisions. As I listened, I became more and more aware that these experts were dealing not with people but with ideas. Nurses deal with people first and use ideas to guide their interactions. One speaker suggested that we might need to start studying what people's experiences are during these high-technology dying processes. He observed this as if no one had ever done so.

I observed that there was a group that had been communicating this very information to groups such as this for years, and were simply dismissed. Nurses, I noted, have never left dying patients and know a great deal about what dying people describe as their experiences. They also know what the families experience. Nurses have told this story in numerous ways, but it has simply not been attended to, having been viewed as less compelling because communicated by a nurse.

The speaker was a bit startled at this idea, seemed to intuitively know it was true, and hurried on to other questions. I was saddened by the response but held my peace and listened more and learned more. Later, several participants approached me and noted that they believed the issue I raised was germane and had given them some new insights into how to approach this difficult issue. I may not have moved the speaker, but I was able to give a few participants a new approach to a troubling idea.

———————

In situations such as this, what often seems apparent to me is that discrimination skills are used largely to shuffle around interesting thoughts in a superficial mind but fail to reach the human dimension, the soul of the human drama. If one introduces these issues of the heart, one risks being dismissed as sentimental. On occasion, however, using careful discrimination skills, one can describe the reality of a human soul, a surer and deeper place, in a knowing way, and evoke new knowing from others and with others. One needs to trust that discrimination can serve intuitive knowing when one chooses to invest in this approach.

Many people who are regularly invited to uneven tables refine and hone their intuitive skills. They tend to need these. They also learn to rely on these skills, since traditional approaches to an uneven table include avoiding any mention of the unevenness. The intuitive hunches about others at the table become gauges for choices made. Trusting one's intuition becomes important because it is often the most reliable source available, especially when no one else at the table is experiencing the unevenness as you are. This reliance on intuition can make efforts at discrimination either seem worthless or farcical. The efforts seem worthless since the skills themselves, applied to realities others deny, are of no utility. The efforts seem like charades, because at an uneven table, those most enthusiastic about discrimination and detail often take this approach to avoid an honest confrontation with more substantive issues.

This leads to an undervaluing of discriminatory skills by those who most need them at an uneven table: those who are disadvantaged. Then, when the skills are most needed, they are like weak and unexercised muscles. They cannot respond to the challenge presented. This is a difficult lesson to learn. Often those who most perceive themselves as victims also choose never to develop these skills, either to avoid self-responsibility or to sustain a process where they can bemoan the fact that they were treated unjustly. Among other things, discriminatory skills help you sort out the pikers from the workers, and help you know who else at the table is working. Workers discriminate, because they know that they need to do so.

One of the important discriminations this unveils is the fact that others at the table experience the same kind of unevenness that you do but may elect to address it in a very different fashion. When you are the sole token unequal participant, this is not a significant issue, but when there are two or more, it adds complexity. Many people at an uneven table will elect to use traditional approaches and invite you to participate. Often others at the table will reward these persons for their "good behavior." Being able to discriminate becomes invaluable in such situations.

Discriminating need not be tedious or odious, but lacks for me the release and freedom of innovation. Hence, I find that I have to be fairly disciplined with myself to pursue it. It helps me to treat it like a course of study, but I find sometimes it feels more like running a gauntlet. I only mention this so that if you feel some distaste bubbling up, you won't have to feel alone. The fact that those you had hoped were your allies are simply practicing their favorite manipulations doesn't help of course, and warrants honest acknowledgment.

Knowing Your Illusions

In addition to assessing the uneven table more precisely, the ability to identify what you do and do not know helps you own your own limitations. The intellectual limits are relatively easy, however, compared to trying to actively own your personal illusions, blindnesses, and distortions. The effort is critical, since these are the very forces that keep you from effective discrimination. The more intimate and personal these illusions, blindnesses, and distortions, the more difficult they are to face and admit, and the more vulnerable they make you at an uneven table. Usually these evoke emotional states, some of which can make you very ineffective at an uneven table. They can also precipitate an escape into shadow projection and its ungainly consequences.

I am often struck by how people who fail to negotiate effectively also refuse to admit basic distortions, blindnesses, and illusions overtly apparent to others. If someone wants to diminish me, and I am busy running away from or denying a basic distortion, blindness, or illusion, it isn't very difficult to find the key to my diminishment. Just touch one of my favorite nerves. That problem, of course, is mine to own, not others'. This seems a very difficult challenge for just about everyone, in my experience. There are choices to be made here.

If indeed I do elect to face and own my own limitations, however, and to confront the ways I distort reality, embrace illusions, or sustain a blindness for whatever reason, I will in time learn that this not only deeply increases my own security, but it also gives me the freedom to ask the same of others. They may not choose to do so, but then the fact that they continue to look through cloudy lenses is public and is theirs to own. It can no longer be used to confuse negotiation.

It is sometimes tempting to fudge on this issue, to think that compassion means distorting truth to fit others' distortions. It takes time and wisdom to learn that once I am enmeshed in another's illusions, I am no longer able to sustain a negotiation, since the illusion controls the process. We are so busy honoring the illusion that truth telling disappears. If I consent to a blindness, I have to spend my time making sure I don't mention the obvious, which is invisible to someone else by choice. If I pretend I see the same distortion as others do, I not only lose my own integrity but fail to present an alternate view that might mitigate the blindness.

There is of course a deep insult embedded in "going along" with another person's illusions, blindnesses, and distortions. I am usually saying that I don't care for you enough to confront these or that I like to use them to manipulate you. There is an ugly cruelty embedded in this process. It may appear to be a comfort but is in the end destructive. This is a hard lesson to learn, since many people do not thank you warmly when you refuse to go along, or conversely, show deep gratitude when you do go along. They may also tell you that this is of no consequence. All illusions are of consequence; all distortions threaten clarity; all blindnesses knowingly maim the truth. These are hard sayings, but ignoring them is worse.

It is important to know, however, the degree to which your invitation to confront limitations has been accepted. People may tell you to quit mentioning their illusions, to ignore their distortions, to leave their blindnesses alone. They may elect to neither confront these themselves nor permit you to acknowledge them. If this occurs, you know a great deal and will need to more actively attend to your personal integrity. The possibility for being a truth teller, even a compassionate truth teller, is significantly diminished and will have a pervasive effect on outcomes. To pretend otherwise is to deny your own reality.

These are demanding activities, however, and require attention, focus, energy, and commitment. If you choose to merely adapt, superficially going along because you are careless about knowing what you do and do not know, you will later find yourself in a morass of distortions you cannot embrace and outcomes you cannot accept. Clarity is difficult, but it is not optional.

Learning

Since the dominant paradigm, carried to its logical limits, denies a substantial portion of reality, those who operate outside the paradigm often find themselves working so hard to sustain their sense of these other realities that they may distort or misunderstand the various positions of people who think and act from the dominant paradigm. To address this, it helps if you don't shy away from being taught. To understand is not to concur. You can learn actively, without being defensive, and in the process discover what others know. Then your anxiety can diminish—not because you are busy protecting your little picture of reality, but because you know not only your reality but something of others' at the table. You can use this information to create innovations. It may help you draw your line in the sand. And of course, you always know that the table is uneven, which is a distinct advantage.

Faking it rarely works, and I personally wouldn't encourage it. If you don't know something, say so. Create an "adult learner" commitment, and live by it. Tell people that you are always out there trying to learn. Most people like to teach others their worldview. Having learned this, you now have access to greater understanding. Sometimes it may even give you access to greater compassion. In this manner, you can gradually reframe "not knowing" so that it becomes an opportunity rather than a threat. You can also create an environment where "willingness to learn" can become a norm rather than an admission of weakness or vulnerability. Under such conditions, everyone can grow. Others might in the process learn more of your worldview, and together the people at the table might craft wiser solutions to their common goals.

Knowing what you do and do not know is more complex than it looks at first, and more demanding. For just that reason, it also has more capacity to make a difference. Neglecting it can make a difference you will rue, and attending to it actively, deliberately, will often make a difference you can celebrate.

An Exercise

One of the most difficult things about this way of being at an uneven table is honest self-appraisal. Most of the time, we like to think of ourselves as pretty open people, learning and growing. We are loathe to describe ourselves as close-minded, fixated on our own viewpoints, stuck in our own little rut. It doesn't even sound nice.

The reality, of course, is that most of us spend quite a bit of time each day finding evidence to support what we already believe, cherish, desire, and defend. We would like to be right more than we would like to be open. Thus, we may seem to be attempting to learn from others, but we are actually listening to them to find where they are correct in their thinking because they think just like we do. In the main, we are not in search of dissonance.

This exercise gives you a chance to begin an honest self-appraisal of the degree to which you are really open and learning, knowing what you do not know and trying to learn about it. It is longer than the other exercises, so you have to make a commitment to do it for one week. I did warn you that this way of being requires discipline, however, so you shouldn't be surprised.

Every night before you retire, for one week, look back over your day and recall the various events and activities. Now write down briefly everything "new" you learned that day. This need only be a few words and should include who you learned it from. Try to list all these events so that you have a comprehensive, one-week record. Do not exclude any examples, and do not form any judgments about the learning sources or content. Just record them factually.

At the end of the week, look over your list for themes. Are there certain people you learn from consistently, or people with certain characteristics: age, gender, ethnicity, proximity? Are there certain kinds of things you seem to learn more readily? Study these patterns for a while. It will of course be comforting to know that you are still open to learning. You may even congratulate yourself a bit on this.

The last part of the exercise is the most interesting. What topics don't appear on your list? Are there people with certain characteristics who never appear on your list? What does this mean? Why is this true? As you answer these last questions, you begin to learn a good deal more about your ability to actually know what you do and do not know.

25

Way of Being Number Nine

Stay in the Dialogue

T his seems pretty obvious, but if you're not at the table, you
can't change anything. You have to be there to make a difference. This is not necessarily good news, however. Over the years, I
have sometimes grown very tired of being at uneven tables, and it
is easy for me to try to make excuses, to try to avoid the patronizing tones, the distortions of my reality, the dismissal of my insights.
The temptation is to absent myself forever. Once I acknowledged
how fruitless and useless traditional approaches to uneven tables
really were, it became even more difficult to continue to show up
at them. I was heartened to learn that more creative ways of being
at such tables exist but also found myself often struggling with the
question of whether I really wanted to continue to show up. These
ways of being are all well and good, but they can prove demanding,
fatiguing, and sometimes painful.

Reframing Time

This way of being addresses the set of disturbing sensations just mentioned. It is a reframe of sorts. The purveyors of the dominant paradigm often define their linear, causal world in a fairly lockstep
fashion: this is the conflict, here are the players, here is the table, we
have two hours to solve this, commence. The emphasis is on getting
control of the situation, usually promptly. Time is treated like a blood

supply: limited, running out. Everything can easily become urgent. The good news is that you need not concur with this judgment.

If the issue were simply control over others, then perhaps this logic would have some validity. If the issues are more compelling, arising from a surer and a deeper place, then conflicts not only need not be solved in one sitting but usually cannot be solved in one sitting. The urgency is often a ploy to rush the process so that no substantive change emerges, so that dominant control is sustained. To address this imposition of urgency is important. You need not define the process as inherently urgent. You can and must be willing to take time-outs, even ones lasting months or years.

This does not, however, mean that you have to leave the dialogue. It is important to be clear that you choose to stay in the dialogue but that you need a time-out. The dialogue about substantive issues will not disappear in your absence. It will wait for you. This is hard work. You will sometimes need to rest. You will need to take care of yourself. If you have been injured, you will need to allow time for healing. These are dimensions of showing compassion for yourself, and they cannot be neglected.

Persons who have spent many hours at uneven tables struggle with these dictums. Often the compelling problems seem to keep you at the table when you know you are now too injured, tired, or impatient to function effectively. You can then become a deterrent rather than a constructive force for change and growth. At such times, stubbornly staying at the table benefits no one. It is thus important to learn that taking a time-out does not mean that you have left the dialogue, but only that you are at this time in retreat.

It is important to beware of people who like to have you at the table to do what they refuse to do, to tell the truths while they risk nothing, to show compassion when they want to hate, to draw the line in the sand without cruelty, to lead the search for a surer and deeper place. They don't want to be at the table alone, or they don't want to be at the table without you there to do for them what they might best learn to do for themselves. If you need a time-out, their pleas are often merely guilt inducing and serve no constructive purpose. Encourage them to try all the things you have modeled for them. Let them own their refusal to risk. If you need the time-out, take it. And assure everyone that you are still in the dialogue.

Discovering Endless Opportunities

It is important to remember that if one goes to an uneven table addressing issues of inequity, attempting to move beyond the mere shuffling of packets of dominant power, there are hundreds of opportunities available to do this. You can find other places, tables, and persons where you can stay creatively in the dialogue. Knowing that the issues are important to you but the tables are multiple and varied is very clarifying. It is an option those invested in controlling others rarely exercise, since the others they focus on tend to be at one specific table.

This changing of tables is an important issue. If you need to change tables, do so. Recognize that if a given table is hopeless, this is not a reason to leave the dialogue but a reason to find a new table. It helps to have a wide-angle lens on reality when you do this. You can more readily recognize a new table when you see it. It also helps if you have developed the ability to trust tomorrow to bring you to another table and another dialogue. Issues of justice don't dissolve themselves. They are also not confined to a single location. If the larger issues capture your attention, there will be tables to sit at for your entire lifetime.

Acknowledging Mobility

The inability to change tables is instructive and merits careful self-assessment, as well as an assessment of others. Some conflicts are sustained precisely because all parties at the table have determined that this is the only available table and that they must prevail. If this is the case, the process actually becomes a long-term dominant power struggle posing as a negotiation. Once I declare that this is the only table I can or will sit at, I effectively commit myself to risking involvement in a destructive or stagnant negotiation. If I remove the possibility of my mobility, I tell everyone else at the table that they ultimately can control me and my integrity, since I will stay no matter what the cost. People at an uneven table often make this mistake, I believe, and then wonder why the outcomes are so troublesome.

The capacity to discriminate between staying in the dialogue and staying in a given negotiation at a given table is imperative if you want to manifest the other ways of being at an uneven table. Those who trusted your commitment at an uneven table need to know that the commitment to the issues persists but the arena may and could change. I need not stay at this one dear table, bludgeoning or being bludgeoned, to demonstrate my commitment to my surer and deeper place. I can go to a new table. It is important and instructive, however, to always assure people clearly that you are still in the dialogue. It can sometimes help those disadvantaged at the table that you are leaving.

Meditation to a Candle Flame

I have no tribe.
You seem to grant this thought
as true, summoned by
my modest act to gain
some small inclusion
in the common fire.

You are my ritual.
You do not send me dogma,
crush desire,
or call for acts of fealty.
You do not ask of me

potato salad in the basement,
coins in the compulsive basket,
passed hand to hand.
You ask no lies.

You start slight fragile,
grow steady, and if I wait,
will beam high enough to
frame my passion,
flame my hopes.

This space and place apart
becomes because of you,
and though communal by your cause,
reminds me of communions of design,
spins me pondering to that precipice
I leaped,
rekindling jagged questions,
still engaging doubts.

In your flicker
I could craft speckled notes
to memory, return.

Your dappling glow
does not permit such sweet meanderings.
Moth-like, I stay the course.
I keep some soft fidelities.

　　—pbk

The decision to stay in the dialogue is actually a question of principle. You do not stay because you are "winning" or leave because you are "losing." The dialogue itself is often the issue, and keeping the conversation going may do more to substantively enhance compassion and increase your capacity to be a truth teller than any gains or losses you may believe have occurred within the dialogue. If you make a commitment to a conversation, it is often a simple conviction about integrity that keeps you in the dialogue. It is also a simple conviction about integrity that may require you to leave a specific table as inappropriate for that dialogue.

Recognizing Interdependence

All major belief systems posit in some fashion the profound inter-dependence of all creatures, of all that we know as our universe. We are all parts or dimensions of a web of life. All conflicts confront us with the fragmentation of that web of relatedness. The fragmenta-tion can worsen, the consequences harm and destroy. The path to war is sometimes very short.

The process of dialogue unveils for us the myriad connections among us; it sensitizes us to their presence, their nature, and their power in our lives. Thus, staying in the dialogue is ultimately a deci-sion to take care of and sustain these connections. They are always more significant and powerful to humans than our conflicts. Our conflicts often fizzle out to some embarrassing inanity. Our connec-tions always have the power to enrich and strengthen us.

Feuds fascinate me sometimes. It is difficult for me to understand why anyone would want to feed one. They are overtly stultifying and lead to chronic fatigue and stagnation. While I can understand the fear beneath them, they seem very contrary to the richness of life and fullness of potential. Thus, staying in our dialogues, all of them, promises more and delivers more to everyone. It takes energy to sustain a dialogue, but it also takes energy to sustain a feud. I can absent myself, but this merely leads to lethargy, inertia, and the death of the human spirit. The dialogue is demanding, but it enlivens more. Despair is always an option, of course, but without substance or the creative potential that hope activates.

Making a commitment to staying in the dialogue is no small issue and merits reflective consideration. It does make demands. That is why compassion for oneself and others is so powerful, why taking the time-outs we need is so imperative, why healing is so significant. It is important to be firm and decisive about staying in the dialogue, but it is equally important to be fluid and flexible in the way we choose to live out that commitment to ourselves and to others, the sites we select or avoid for our commitments. An example may be helpful.

A Story

Perhaps no force in my career has harmed nurses as much as the women's movements. This has been painful for me to confront, since I am deeply committed to the balancing of the forces of masculine and feminine principle in our culture, and indeed on our planet. For most of my career, I have supported women's issues and have found this anomalous situation vexing.

When the women's movements of the seventies emerged, they often focused on the rights of women to have access to career opportunities traditionally discouraged for women, if not actually withheld. One of these was medicine, and the conviction was that to seek equality was to seek access to medical education. In a strange twist of reasoning, this was presented not as the opportunity for freedom of choice, but the right to become a powerful, high-status physician rather than being forced to be a powerless, low-status nurse. A whole generation of young women, including my own daughters, were immersed in this worldview.

This distortion was destructive to all nurses and all young men and women who might have been attracted to nursing. Our nursing school enrollments plummeted, and many who enrolled in nursing schools came either with apologies for having failed to choose medicine or with a deep conviction that their powerlessness and worthlessness might make them good nurses. The eighties were laced for me with these experiences and with the damage done to the nurses who we will want to care for us someday. Declining enrollments continue to this day, portending the most serious nursing shortage of my career.

In addition, growing numbers of young women sought what was held out to them as a superior choice and became physicians, but with the clear understanding that they had avoided the tragedy of being a nurse. These women too were harmed, and in turn harmed many nurses. It was, and continues to be, a very destructive process. It seemed more and more to me to be a situation where the hatred of women for women took a particularly virulent turn.

Intellectually, I could reason that oppressed people often turn on their own, that nurses were for many men and women the personification of the women created by the dominant paradigm. For many, our work appears to be archetypally female work. Most saw us coopted. Few realized that negotiating with a physician hierarchy and still doing much good was an amazing achievement. When they saw us accommodate physicians who behaved in destructive ways toward us, they rarely recognized that we often accommodated this behavior with considerable insight and did so to protect or help patients, many of whom trusted these physicians and would have been harmed had that trust been damaged. The inability to imagine our awareness levels was discouraging.

This was for me a critical challenge in my effort to stay in the dialogue, to find tables where I could continue to support the growing voice of women, yet refuse to compromise my integrity by negating nurses. It required compassion with just about everyone and often a decision to leave a table committed to sustaining the distortion. Although I am not a patient woman, it has called forth from me more patience than I thought I possessed. It has also asked of me a courage to keep some fidelity to nurses despite all the invitations to participate in the societal negation of nurses.

The complex efforts, the need to take time-outs and heal, the willingness to stay in the dialogue and to leave tables I must leave, and the decision to yet once more try to be the truth teller have been challenging. It has been particularly difficult to listen to young women physicians explain to me that they at first considered being a nurse, but then realized that they wanted to ask more of themselves than merely being a nurse. Such physicians, like most, have little knowledge or awareness of how "unmerely" being a nurse really is. To stay in the dialogue under these tough conditions is for me my life exemplar of this way of being.

In the effort to stay in the dialogue, confusion can emerge about precisely what the dialogue is all about. The most compelling human issues involve dialogue about our connectedness. It is clear that for all of us, conflict visits our lives and alters our sense of well-being. That conflict tends to be with other humans. We need to remember too, however, that the most moving dimensions of being human also occur with other humans. If we seek to be with other humans, we risk conflict. The hard work of slogging through these conflicts is a facet of human experience and human relatedness.

To struggle toward a surer and deeper place where we try to grasp and solve our conflicts involves us in more complex and fulfilling relationships with others. Then conflict becomes not a deterrent or a tragedy, but an opportunity for growth and self-realization. The conflict-free relationship is an illusion and at best indicates stagnation, suppression, or denial. Thus, if we want more from life, we will need to relate, and if we relate, we will experience conflict. Staying in the dialogue says that we want this fulfillment and are willing to do the work of conflict resolution to achieve our goal.

Since much conflict resolution focuses on a fixation with dominant power, it is critical to ascertain the likelihood of any given table shifting from a rigid position. If there is little chance of this happening, one is not in a dialogue. Indeed, most conflict resolution rituals that fixate on this level are adversarial in tone and are so common in our culture that they often appear to be—or even are—scripted. Two overt examples of this are courtroom proceedings and union negotiations, where an array of "customary" practices have emerged to keep the level fixed and the participants fixated.

A Story

Few human experiences equal the wrenching and painful nature of divorce. Yet it is an experience many people in the United States have, and one that is rendered far more destructive because of the assumption of an adversarial process. When I faced this process, I worked very hard to try to make the experience one that would do as little damage as possible. I was struck, at every turn, by the structures and practices in place that assumed the process would be adversarial and that actually encouraged and rewarded adversarial behavior.

There were many experiences along the road to the courtroom, but I was still not prepared to deal with a judge worried about my unwillingness to behave in an adversarial fashion. Having sworn me in as a witness to the proceedings, he asked me if I didn't want a provision in the final divorce decree that permitted me to come back to court if some tragedy befell me and I then wanted my former husband to assist me. He was concerned that I had not included this provision and pressed me to request it. I said I did not want this provision.

He became belligerent with me. "So who do you think is going to take care of you if something happens?" he asked angrily. I answered that I had friends and family who would come to my aid. "You'd be surprised how everyone will abandon you when you're in trouble," he responded, and then announced that I clearly had not thought this over carefully enough and so he was unwilling to grant the divorce. Our lawyer asked for a recess, and after an hour of waiting, he reopened our case.

When I returned to the stand, he insisted that I enter a statement into the court record that said I wanted the provision he had insisted on. I responded that I wanted this because he would otherwise not grant my divorce. This did not please him. It was his conviction that I had to say I wanted it myself. Realizing that we were locked in a conflict where each of us chose to stay on very different levels of discourse, I consented to his statement.

Reflecting back on this judge's well-intentioned but disturbing behavior, I realized that his worldview assumed an adversarial process, and since I was not behaving in an adversarial fashion, I had no doubt failed to understand the seriousness of my decision. As a result, he decided, I had not been provided with adequate protections, and in his kindness, he hoped to assure me of these. The fact that I did not want his protections simply proved to him how uninformed I was.

Fixated dialogues are not really dialogues, but repetitive scripts. It is important to make this distinction, since staying in a repetitious script is self-defeating and dangerous, a far cry from staying in a dialogue. This way of being at an uneven table only makes sense if you can assure yourself that you are in a dialogue. Knowing the levels of discourse that you wish to live on is thus critical. Once you know these levels, you can better ascertain which tables you are willing to go to, and what dialogues you choose to sustain.

Not only is it useful to know if others at a table are fixated; it is equally important to determine if you yourself are fixated. Some people go to a table not to create, but merely to express their anger and vengeance about the problem of uneven tables. They do not wish to resolve conflicts but merely to unveil the disaster of the uneven table. Often they don't really want the table to become even, since they get a great deal of satisfaction out of harping about the uneven table.

A bit of self-assessment is in order to determine if this is the case. If you are often invited to uneven tables and you have grown weary of the process, you can easily fixate on this: "Oh no, not another uneven table!" That is why it is important to take timeouts and heal as needed. If you become driven, you become ineffective. You also can become attached to the secondary gains of being the hard-driving or tragic creature who keeps showing up at uneven tables. I find it helps me a great deal in this regard to make sure I have many dialogues where being even is valued and getting even is not a goal. It heightens my reality-testing skills, and it comforts me.

An Exercise

The quickest way to determine your own behavior in relation to staying in the dialogue is to watch and observe your own patterns. As you've read this book, you have recorded several conflicts or negotiations or both. You actually should have an ample collection by now. Return to your journal and flip through it. Find the examples you've recorded thus far. As you find one, study it a while. Then answer the following questions.

Did the conflict get resolved? If so, did it or a related one recur with this person or group? If so, did you return to the individuals involved and try to seek a resolution? If not, why not? Would you consider trying to do so now? What would you do differently? Are some of these conflicts you hope to never revisit? Why?

As you review each recorded conflict and answer questions, it is often helpful to begin watching for the conflicts you return to and the ones you abandon unresolved. After you have answered the questions about each, you can then search for the pattern. In your journal, take a single page and draw a line down the middle. On one side, give brief characteristics of the conflicts or negotiations you returned to. On the other side, give the same brief characteristics of ones you did not return to.

After you have done this with all the conflicts you can find lurking in your journal, reflect on the two columns a bit. What do the conflicts in each column have in common? Most of us stay in some dialogues more readily than others. If you can find some common patterns in those you leave, you can begin to find out where and how you elect to not stay in the dialogue. These will often be the most challenging conflicts, and therefore the ones most likely to increase your skill and growth. Hence, the very dialogues you do not stay in are often your best opportunity for creative self-enhancement. You may want to reconsider your willingness to persistently walk away from these opportunities.

———————

26

Way of Being Number Ten
Know When and How to Leave the Table

You may have noticed that all along I've been mentioning that you might actually leave the table. This last way of being addresses that possibility and brings together the other ways of being. By now you have hopefully noticed that they are all interdependent, just like I promised. If you let one go awry, others will often follow and will always be maimed or tainted. They depend on one another.

All of them depend somewhat uniquely on this one, and this one depends somewhat uniquely on each of the others. You may recall that very early I told you the story about claimers and creators. The ways of being are about being creative, even if you are at an uneven table. Sometimes, however, you find that someone at the table is hell bent on claiming, and there is nothing to be done about it.

This is almost always the easiest situation to identify when you are trying to determine if you need to consider leaving the table. Claimers persist, and never do get to any creative agenda, so they are relatively easy to locate. Some claimers, however, when questioned, will tell you that they are creators. Then you will need to make an independent judgment. They will repeatedly tell you that they are working very hard to get beyond claiming and to engage in creating. They may tell you this often, for weeks, months, and years. In such situations, the claimers' responses to the other nine ways of being at an uneven table are useful guides.

Claimers must prevail. They need to win. They need their worldview to prevail. They need to be proven right. These needs are often veiled. Others at the table may not even recognize a claimer when they see one. A very skillful claimer can manipulate the process without revealing these needs and yet get them met. Claimers often embrace the dominant paradigm. You may find yourself at a table where everyone is so accustomed to seeing the dominant paradigm as the only valid worldview that no one notices all the claiming going on. People may simply see this as normal or inevitable.

Some people at the table may have found ways to get an array of secondary gains by keeping the claimer "happy." They may benefit personally from covertly controlling the claimer, from manipulating the claimer. They may have created a dependency in the claimer for self-aggrandizement or egocentricity and may use this dependency to achieve their ends. Often the traditional ways of being at an uneven table are so entrenched that virtually no one else at the table can imagine an alternative. They are also unwilling to change this reality because they can't imagine better outcomes than the ones they have settled for.

The interdependence of the ten ways of being at an uneven table can prove invaluable in such situations. Each of the first nine ways provides you with a database for decision making, tells you whether this indeed is a table where you should continue to sit, helps you know when you should leave the table. Hence, to access the tenth way of being, the most trustworthy approach is to make manifest the other nine ways and observe the outcomes.

When you attempt to invite the participants in a conflict to go to a surer and deeper place, the response to the invitation becomes information you need if you are making a decision to leave or stay. If you suggest that we might want to remember what is best for our children or our children's children and a participant tells you we don't need to get all mushy about children since we're dealing with hard, cold facts here, you need to observe this person closely. He or she may be telling you that the process will fixate at a single level and will not move. If the level is one of sustaining the conflict, or of one party prevailing, this is not a table you would choose to stay at. It is important to recall at this point that claimers always win, and by staying at the table, you participate in the outcomes of the negotiation, and thus give tacit consent to these outcomes.

Most people intuitively are attracted to going to a surer or deeper place and may thus accept your invitation initially. As the negotiation progresses, they may discover that the surer deeper place asks them to make choices, to release old habits or seeming advantages that they are loathe to surrender. They may stay in the surer deeper place for a while and then suddenly bolt. It is important to watch for this departure. While you may regret it, or it may sadden you, the fact that it happens is significant. Once people leave the surer deeper place, the negotiation will shift dramatically and you may find yourself at a table where leaving is your wisest next transaction.

Truth telling often reveals an analogous response. If persons at the table actively silence you, or tell you that your observations are not germane to the topic, or that you should not be bringing up these issues that upset everyone, you have an indicator that the negotiation may not be authentic. If selected truths are to be systematically denied and you believe these to be central to the conflict, the silencing or dismissal of these truths would indicate that this is not a table you wish to remain at.

Here again, you may find that persons at the table initially commit to truth telling. Then, abruptly, some truth emerges that they had hoped to ignore, deny, or distort. Suddenly, after much progress, the negotiation shifts from resolving the conflict to silencing the truth that will not be confronted. This can be quite confusing and requires reflective, focused attention. The most readily available indicator is that there will now be clear boundaries about what may or may not be said. When some truths become persistently and systematically forbidden, the table has changed and you may need to walk away.

At some juncture in most negotiations, you will discover that people will offer you an invitation to "sell your soul"—that is, they will ask you to no longer honor your integrity. While you may elect to clearly do otherwise, it is important to ascertain just what this invitation is communicating and how often it is made. It is also useful to determine the actual focus of the invitation, what particular dimension of your soul people want you to sell. While the most overt offer may focus on moral integrity, such persons may also be willing to put a price on intellectual or spiritual or emotional integrity. This teaches you both something about yourself and something about the table. A table that persistently or even frequently implies that you need not honor your integrity is one that may prove, over time, to be pursuing goals you cannot embrace. If others at the table fail to honor their integrity, this too can serve as an indicator. Once integrity is compromised, it can become a virtual epidemic, and leaving before the infection spreads may be a critical turning point in the negotiation.

This indicator has proven particularly useful for me. While I may stay for a time at a table that neglects or undervalues my integrity or that of others, a norm is being set and sustained that gives a clue to the types of outcomes that may emerge from the negotiation. I may very successfully honor my integrity and yet find that since personal integrity is not a serious value of the participants, a solution to a conflict will be crafted that seems to honor my integrity but neglects that of others. Since I am party to this process, it has then failed to honor mine.

A Story

As academic communities in the United States have become more and more captivated by the value framework of the dominant paradigm, the intrusion of a discipline such as nursing into these enclaves has often been resisted. While nursing embraces much of the dominant paradigm, it does so only with an equal commitment to the value framework of the emerging paradigm. It is also an almost exclusively female discipline. These characteristics have made it often seem out of sync with traditional academic norms.

Nowhere has this resistance been felt as keenly as in the effort to develop and implement doctoral programs in nursing. If indeed nurses and women cannot be viewed as equal partners in the academic community, it is clearly unrealistic to assume they might develop rigorous and competent programs of study leading to the awarding of doctoral degrees.

One of the ways nursing faculties have dealt with this is to meet the requirements of the academy with a frenzy—to go above and beyond the minimal expectations in an effort to demonstrate competence and parity. This has been a demanding process and is sometimes irksome, but the gains in strength and capacity have been valuable. Nurses know that they will only achieve this goal if they walk straight up a very perpendicular mountain. Rather than complaining about the injustice, they simply go out and buy high-quality hiking gear.

The first doctoral program I developed endured this process. As a result, the final proposal was unanimously approved by an initially skeptical campus community. In seeking approval from state educational leaders, however, the process turned political, and feelings ran high. As the person attempting to negotiate this process, I found on one side a frustrated and angry nursing community that had waited far too long for equity in educational opportunity. On the other was a reluctant group of educational administrators. In good faith, I kept all their rules, honored all their requests and demands, and asked my colleagues to do likewise, to negotiate in good faith.

During these negotiations, however, I was offered several strange options, all of which would have disadvantaged or diminished one or another nursing group in the state. In essence, I was being told that if I was willing to harm another group of nurses, I would indeed have an approved doctoral program. While I recognized the invitation to compromise my integrity and chose not to do so, I also learned from these invitations that I was negotiating at a table where integrity was not a value.

Eventually, I realized that these negotiations were not sincere and that this was a table I needed to leave. In doing so, I first informed the administrators involved that I no longer believed we were engaged in a good-faith negotiation. I then no longer discouraged my colleagues from expressing their anger and frustration, and a fairly intense wave of political pressure emerged, which resulted in the approval of the program but in the end did not benefit the educational administrators.

Had they honored my integrity, they might have negotiated their way to a more creative resolution. It was instructive to me that they were unable to imagine that nurses seeking a goal with tenacity and honesty would be taken seriously. Since they did not take the dreams and hopes and wishes of nurses seriously, they assumed others, including nurses, would do the same. The lesson was a costly one for them, both in political outcomes and in personal integrity.

Over the years, I have found this touchstone of personal integrity the most valuable tool for me in evaluating uneven tables. It takes people to the heart of the matter quickly and efficiently. We who have spent much of our careers at uneven tables often have little else beyond our integrity when we leave the table, so it is critical to me that this at least I have in tow as I walk away. Hence, invitations to dirty deals are always a sign to me that the table is not one where I choose to continue to search for surer and deeper places to address issues of concern to me. Over time I have also learned that those accustomed to exercising dominant power tend to assume that disadvantaged persons will accept dirty deals, and are often confused or enraged when the deal is refused. Moral agency is not an expectation.

Inviting compassion to the table can also provide useful information about the table, and whether you wish to remain at it. If compassion is unseated, invited to leave, or never permitted a seat, the outcomes of the conflict may have the same character: compassionless. While many conflicts have solutions that attend poorly to compassion, I have found that these kinds of solutions are often expedient and in the end do more harm than good. They look good at first but later create further disasters.

It is perhaps obvious that if you draw a line in the sand and people at the table do not accept this line, you need to leave. That is why it is so helpful to draw the line early. If it is intolerable to parties to the conflict, you already know that you probably shouldn't stay. You may simply waste your time and energy redrawing a line folks keep on erasing. If you have to draw your line in the sand over and over again, you are not engaging in a negotiation but a new power struggle about your right to have a line in the sand.

As becomes apparent, all these dynamics tend to interact. They are often mitigated, however, by efforts to expand and explicate the context and to innovate. If parties to a conflict are willing to engage in these two activities, they can sometimes see their way to surer and deeper places, truth telling, integrity, and compassion. This will not always be the case but does occur often enough that you need to weigh this potential against resistances to other ways of being. Sometimes compassion or truth telling becomes the innovation, or the surer and deeper place becomes the new context. These two ways of being thus serve to provide some balance to the impact of the earlier ways of being and help demonstrate why all ten together work synergistically.

The progression through a negotiation is improved through the process of knowledge sharing. As this unfolds, your level of preparedness is critical, and if it is inadequate, you may be at a table you are not yet knowledgeable enough to handle. This may injure your pride a bit, but it is an important issue to address. If you do not have the knowledge you need to stay at the table, it is wiser by far to simply leave and get the knowledge you need. You may also determine to stay long enough to see if you can acquire the knowledge while you are at the table, but it has been my experience that this is risky and needs to be done sparingly. If you lack knowledge, even if you are a quick learner, outcomes may be crafted that include dimensions that you do not understand; had you understood them, you might not have accepted them.

The ninth way of being actually focuses on what you can do if you indeed must leave a given table. It gives you the option to continue to embrace your goals but still holds you to leaving a specific table you discover is unacceptable to you. It thus assists you in a meaningful and constructive exit and helps you frame for yourself a way to address the impact of this departure.

Knowing the Evolutionary Moment

As you can see, the ways of being at the table are invaluable in helping you know when to leave. For that reason, it is important to collect the other nine ways when you leave a table and to clearly explain to others at the table that you are leaving and that you are taking these ways with you. Whenever possible, it is helpful to those you leave behind if you clearly explain why you are leaving. As you leave, try to remember that there are thousands of other tables and that in seating yourself at these, you continue to create the future.

Ultimately, leaving a table is about change. It stems from a sensitivity to the evolutionary moment, both for you and for others. The only real evolutionary moment you control is your own; the only real change you can effect is the change you effect within yourself. You can create the conditions for others to change and evolve, but this ensures nothing. You do not control others' choices about change. You do not control their evolutionary moments.

It is important to be rigorously honest with yourself about the absence of change. Life is change, and the absence of change is an indicator of stagnation, fixation, and in some cases a form of "death." If you are negotiating at a table where no change occurs, you may have become part of a process of stagnation. Your presence may even sustain the stagnation. Often this stagnation is simply the persistent fixation on a claiming process among parties jockeying for dominance power. It is important to realize that this is no longer a negotiation. It is a competition. If virulent, it is a war.

Since I have often been an outspoken person, I have found myself at some tables where the illusion of negotiation was being sustained by pointing out that I was present, and that proved something must be happening. This is a sophisticated version of cooptation. It can also be used by others to absent themselves from the costs of participation.

Self-indulgence, laziness, and hopelessness all are forces that can keep us at a table we should leave, one where we know that the negotiation has gone stale, that change is not possible, that we are collectively stuck and unable to unfreeze ourselves. It is important to remember in such situations that not deciding to leave is in itself a decision. Sometimes vanity keeps us from these hard choices, or our own deep stubbornness, or our fear of others' reactions. It is difficult to confront these messier, darker dimensions of our decision making, but to fail to do so is even more difficult once the consequences begin to unfold. Shadow work emerges whether invited or not.

Caring About Our Self-Worth

Decisions about leaving tables are often decisions about our own self-worth. If we have a limited opinion of ourselves, we may be willing to stay at just about any table and hang out there looking like we're busy doing something with our lives. We may go through the charades or sustain an illusion because we are too cowardly to strike out on a new path. We may not want to face our own truths or admit that we made a mistake and went to the wrong table to start with. We live in a culture that often says staying is a virtue, but we need to discriminate carefully, to know what we're choosing and why. If we're not part of a solution to a problem, we are then probably part of the problem itself.

If I stay because others assure me that I should or that they want me there, I need to determine the degree to which these messages preserve or damage my personal integrity. I also need to honestly confront my own desire to gain acceptability at the cost of that integrity. Others may simply want me to stay to help them avoid their own hard choices. Staying is sometimes merely self-destruction, and modeling it for others may support their self-destruction. Finding your courage and facing your own cowardice may also assist others in doing the same.

Owning Your Refusals

If you refuse to leave a table you should leave, if you refuse to move to new realities when you know that you cannot sustain the ways of being at the one where you're now seated, it is critical that you own this decision. It is always tempting to blame others for this refusal to try a new venue: "Oh, they need me so much"; "I was so vital to their process"; "They could not do it without me"; "They depended on me"; "I didn't want to disappoint them. . . ." This list can get fairly long. It sounds positive, but it is merely a list of excuses that blame and project. The reason you fail to leave a table that you know you should leave is because you lack imagination and courage. This is your problem, not anyone else's.

Leaving tables is always difficult, but it is even more difficult to stay where you know you don't belong. When you are seated at an uneven table, you know that you started the process with participants who accepted the inequity. They may choose not to change. This is their right. Your unwillingness to accept this fact is your problem, not theirs. If you value your own worth enough, if you recognize the fact that you have something important to bring to conflict resolution, you will not waste your time and energy on people who have made a commitment to staying locked into ways of being that you do not embrace.

Hence, leaving the table can also prove to be an act of self-worth and self-affirmation. If you value your life, your energy, your very self, you want to only negotiate at the best of tables. They may still be uneven, but that will always be the case. If they must be uneven, it would be nice if they were at least the best of the lot. It is important to leave with pride and dignity, with graciousness. This helps you focus on the ways of being as you walk toward your next table with hope.

An Exercise

Think of all the tables you've left over the last five years. Write down these situations. A few brief words will do it. Now, beside each, write down why you left the table. Beside each, write yes if you like your reason, no if you didn't. Do this process rapidly, off the top of your head.

Now, take your list of the ten ways of being at an uneven table. Look at each situation more reflectively, and ask yourself how these ten ways apply to that situation. See if you can find something familiar, something congruent. Sometimes we find that we instinctively know that we need to leave but have not yet learned to trust this process. Take some time to give yourself credit for having done so. Where you find reasons you feel less positive about, try to ascertain what was going on with these, and indeed, what is probably still going on for you to this day.

Now, think of two or three conflict situations in your life where you are engaged in ongoing negotiations that are part of your daily life. You might include your boss, or a friend, or a partnership, or an organization you belong to. Perhaps it is a community activity you are taking part in. Look at each situation for a while. Give special attention to any players in the situation who seem to chronically irk or upset you. These provocations are almost always the best place to learn something worthwhile.

Are any of these tables you should leave? Have you tried the other nine ways of being at these tables yet? If you did, what would happen? Would you leave if you needed to do so? If not, why not? What keeps you at tables you should leave? Do you like this part of yourself? Do you want to strengthen this part of yourself? Can you change? Do you want to? What would happen if you did change? It helps here to write down your fears, your vanities, your stubbornness. Are you afraid of what others would think of you, that you might be making a mistake, that you just hate to lose?

Picture yourself leaving these tables. How would you do it? How does it feel? Did you gain or lose in the process? Can you find another place to stay in the dialogue? Are you afraid that you can't? Is this a good enough reason to stay at the table? What do you want to do about all this?

Could leaving the table be an act of liberation, of self-worth, of honesty, of courage, of integrity, of compassion for yourself and others?

What price do you pay for staying at a table you should leave? Is it worth it?

27

Some Antidotes and Precautions

So there you have it, the ten ways of being at an uneven table:

1. *Find and inhabit the deepest and surest human space that your capabilities permit.*

2. *Be a truth teller.*

3. *Honor your integrity, even at great cost.*

4. *Find a place for compassion at the table.*

5. *Draw a line in the sand without cruelty.*

6. *Expand and explicate the context.*

7. *Innovate.*

8. *Know what you do and do not know.*

9. *Stay in the dialogue.*

10. *Know when and how to leave the table.*

Thinking back, you doubtless noticed that they are pretty difficult. I agree. I also know that if you are consistently finding yourself at uneven tables, what you're doing now is pretty difficult. What these ways of being offer you is something difficult that can actually feel better and stands a better chance of making a positive difference for change. To go incessantly to uneven tables is enough of a problem. To go with some new tools and with a sense of evolutionary possibility can only be an improvement.

Getting Perspective

Some precautions are in order. It is critical in using these ways of being that you carefully do your homework intellectually, emotionally, and morally. I have provided one simple exercise with each way of being to give you a chance to focus on this type of homework. It is easy to memorize this list or try to give the appearance of these ways of being. To live them experientially, honestly, and creatively is quite another thing. They all call for a level of courage, for the will and the action that make truth manifest. You can try to fake it, but it won't work.

You may want to use these ways of being to "win" at an uneven table. If that is the case, you may want to reflect on what you really think I said in this book. If I win anything at the expense of another, the victory is inevitably hollow. I may have prevailed, but my humanity will be diminished. That is precisely what has irked you about all those people fixated on dominant power at uneven tables. Why do you want to become one of them? If your goal is vengeance, this is the wrong book for you to have read.

I know this is all pretty blunt and forceful, but I wrote this book carefully, trying to be very clear. I am not interested in helping people act even more weird at uneven tables than they already do now. This book, these ways of being ask a lot of you, but they also give you many more opportunities to grow, to become more whole and more fulfilled.

I do have a good deal of empathy with people who get sick and tired of having to go to uneven tables. I often have the same reaction. When I lose perspective, I try to find it again. Here's how I do that.

An Exercise

Float yourself up to a cloud. I know that sounds strange, but do it anyway, just float yourself up there. This can actually be pretty fun. Sit down, relax, enjoy the view. Pretty panoramic, huh! Now, imagine that since you have this great view of the whole universe, you are not only equipped to see pretty extensively in space, but also in time. Imagine the last two hundred years slowly. Now imagine the next two hundred years. Take as much time as you need. As you may have noticed, what with four hundred years to play with, time is in plentiful supply.

Now, recall yourself at the most recent uneven table you have visited. Ask yourself, here, sitting staring at the whole known universe, at the last and next two-hundred-year time spans, just how important this issue really is. Think about that a while.

Well, eventually you were going to have to come down from the clouds and face the here and now. Welcome back.

Seeking Wisdom

Having gotten a bit more perspective, you can begin to see that your capacity for wisdom might just be worth investing in. All of us are struggling toward more comprehensive capacities for self-responsibility. We all would like to correct some of our mistakes of the past. We all would like to create a better future for our children. Ways of being at an uneven table enable that process.

I think one more story about my daughter Tricia will give you yet another way of imagining the ways of being.

A Story

Early in Tricia's life, it became apparent that she was a person who would achieve academically. Both her curiosity and her natural intelligence were strong, and she had the discipline to follow both. She was easily a teacher's dream come true and steadily progressed in mastering the rituals of the U.S. educational system.

I identified with this trait of Tricia's, and, like many mothers, felt some joy and pride, but also the apprehension that comes with wanting to save your children from the more troublesome dimensions of your own personal history. Hence, I was wary of the strong reinforcement our culture gives a child such as Tricia to focus too much on academic achievement. So many rewards come to one from this dimension that it is easy to become unbalanced.

I worried about this, and sometimes we discussed it in that way children and their mothers craft discussions about complex issues. These discussions could manifest as support of her playful side, or her rich personal character, or her artistic ability, or her athletic skills, but the goal was that she reach her full potential and fulfillment. I was never fully certain if she understood this, though no doubt she sensed the urgency I sometimes inadvertently signaled.

When she was in third grade, her father and I went to one of those parent-night "show and tell" ceremonies. In her school, this involved not only meeting with the teacher individually but also surveying the room for posted projects that all children had done. As usual, Tricia got rave reviews in the individual session with the teacher, and the nervous voice was active in me as we wandered about the room looking at the displays.

On one bulletin board the teacher had hung pictures drawn by all the children in the class. Each child had drawn a picture of what they intended to be as adults. We scanned them, looking for Tricia's. There were the pictures of the "when I grow up I'm going to be an astronaut" and the "when I grow up I'm going to be a ballerina" mixed in with the more modest firemen and stewardesses. The elaborate pictures that accompanied these were a delight.

Then we found Tricia's. Staring back at us was a young woman simply smiling at us. She had no special uniform, no special activity, no special props. Underneath Tricia had printed: "When I grow up, I'm going to be well rounded." We scanned the board. No doubt about it, she was the only kid in the class with this rather unusual goal.

Over the years, as I have watched her receive a variety of awards and recognitions, many of them academic, I have always recalled this picture story. The recall is strongest when I am in a situation where I see the awards, both public and private, she has received for being well rounded and the other awards she forgoes to achieve this. In the tradition of mothers everywhere, I always recall this story to Tricia at such times. I picture her reading it now, saying to herself, "There she goes again!" A good story full of wisdom deserves several tellings, Tricia!

28

A Progress Report

As I noted in the beginning of this edition of *Negotiating at an Uneven Table*, my intent has been to give an update. This update has two sources. The first is the many students and readers who have graciously entered a dialogue with me, and shared both what they have found useful and what they have found unclear or problematic. The second source is far more personal, and involves the lessons about negotiating at an uneven table that I have learned in the intervening years. While I have woven in much of both throughout the book, this chapter addresses these latter lessons more directly.

I suppose I knew at the outset that writing this book was a bit presumptuous of me, a bit harrowing as adventures go. The decision to include a reference to moral courage in the title was a difficult one. And, I was primarily trying to tell my life lessons. Doing so has not become easier. I have been deeply enriched by and benefited from the dialogues and experiences catalyzed by this book. I have also been challenged in ways I would not have imagined.

The greatest challenge for me has been to go more deeply into everything I discussed here, to open myself to learning more profoundly the lessons I described. Looking back in the rearview mirror, I believe that despite my moments of failure, I have succeeded to some degree, and in the process affirmed what I wrote. I find, however, that I want to underline some parts, print them in bold, alert the reader that this or that idea is really very important. I experience this as scope of comprehension seeking voice.

A Story

To share what I have learned, I need to tell yet another story. As with all my stories, it tells only my perspective, the experiences I have had. Others will no doubt tell the story quite differently.

I have a "day job" as a university professor. I was hired, about the time I started writing the first edition of this book, to develop and implement a doctoral program in nursing. I had developed one before, and looked forward to doing so again, incorporating all the things I had learned from making mistakes the first time around. I was enthused and committed.

I had moved to another part of the country, to a new culture. I had been a dean for several years and wanted to return to the life of a professor so that I could spend more time in the work of scholarship and writing. I was now part of a health science center, no longer with easy access to all the other academic disciplines that had always been part of my life and work, catalysts for my imagination. I had left behind a complex, extensive, and affirming support system built over eighteen years. I had left behind familiar cultural mores and practices, ones congruent with my own Midwestern roots.

I had become increasingly focused on better understanding negotiating at an uneven table. It was the focus of my scholarship and writing. Intermittently, I would leave my "day job" to lecture or teach about uneven tables throughout the United States. The hundreds of people I worked with helped me see that explicating this process was important to far more people than I had imagined. The work was gratifying, and helped me to begin development of the book that builds on this one, the book that describes the negotiation skills rarely mastered by people not born to the table.

It took me eight years to understand the relationships between these two activities of creating a doctoral program and learning about negotiation, to understand that more than ever before in my life, I was living at an uneven table on the day job while teaching about it elsewhere. As the table became more uneven, the learning accelerated and deepened.

————————

The work of creating the doctoral program was exciting as we began. The school of nursing where I worked was willing to go through an arduous process of self-examination to devise the best program possible, one that best fit this school, faculty, and traditions. We elected to focus the program on healing as a central nursing construct.

While the decision was made collectively and carefully, over time, none of us had any idea how revolutionary we actually were. No other nursing program anywhere focused on healing. We who work in health care often act as if the only kind of human healing we attend to is physical in nature, and to even use the word healing is somehow a bit too "soft," not the stuff of the "hard" sciences we want health care to exemplify. While we all agree that we are invested in healing, naming it the central focus of a doctoral program was a risk, and took us to places we had not imagined we would visit.

The word *healing*, derived from the Old English word *haelen*, meaning wholeness, refers not only to a desired wholeness, but also to the process of moving toward that desired wholeness, and includes the interactions that lead to that desired wholeness. As the party responsible for leadership in developing the program, I set out in my solid stolid Germanic fashion to become an expert in the concept. If we agreed this was to be our goal, then it seemed imperative that I master the construct as comprehensively as possible. I also set out to collaborate with my faculty colleagues to create a program that would enable our doctoral students to become scholars of the concept, to become experts in the study of healing practices in nursing. What I discovered is that we had committed ourselves as a group to going to a deeper and surer human space than I had ever gone with any group.

Creating a Preferred Future

It was exhilarating. We had collectively shifted. We were actually playing out the balancing act between the dominant and emerging paradigms. We were exploring the sciences that address wholeness. We were both building on the past and creating new futures. We sought wholeness for our students, our program, and ourselves. We were on a new terrain, beyond the dominance power fixation, consciously evolving new ways of knowing and being. We adopted a program philosophy that publicly abandoned the historic power relationships between teacher and student, embracing a partnership of learning. We confronted conflicts; we resolved them. Students flourished, and we flourished with them.

We discovered early on that a clear understanding of healing confronts dominance power. Healers don't heal people. We heal ourselves. Healing is an internal, natural process. We either heal, or we die. What we in health care do is create the conditions that optimize the healing process. That takes the control away from the health care provider, and returns it to the persons seeking healing. They alone can say when what we do is working. They also can interrupt or prohibit their healing, and there is little we can do about this. We health care providers do not control healing; we merely create optimal context and support the process.

The concept of wholeness also confronts multiple ways of knowing. All ways of knowing count when one is searching for wholeness. We even published a book of our reflections on healing, in which forty members of our community shared their understanding of healing in a variety of ways of knowing: poetry, scholarly articles, parables, personal stories (Kritek, 1997). For the first time, in that book I recorded what was for me a growing realization that negotiation was a healing practice. As the book's editor, I was moved by the richness of perspective, the courage of the authors, the blending of dominant and emerging paradigms in print. I would often refer to it as a quilt of women's voices.

As I noted here at the outset, no doubt others would tell a different story of these events. I of course am telling my story, the one I experienced.

Return to the Uneven Table

As the program grew, we evaluated the components of the program needing amplification or refinement. We knew we needed to expand our faculty numbers to meet student interest in the program, an interest greater than we had at first imagined. We also began to notice that living in the deepest and surest space was demanding. Not everyone enjoyed it, and old familiar patterns beckoned. The comfort of social congruence diminished, the further we progressed. And many people, schooled as women in the South, missed manipulation when the conflicts emerged. Old patterns of conflict avoidance steadily reasserted themselves. I, the Yankee, no doubt often missed the cues of this reassertion.

We had found our way to a new paradigm, but also realized that we had not yet fully integrated the voice of the dominant paradigm. Intellectual integrity required that this voice be heard and integrated into the whole. We set out to ensure that it would. We had perhaps forgotten, however, that this voice must prevail, must win, claims at any cost, seeks prediction and control. We invited it to the table, and asked it to be just another voice. That of course was not congruent with its sense of entitlement. Inadvertently, we had reactivated the uneven table so familiar to us all. Wholeness called for this voice; the voice itself was eager to silence all others.

Negotiations were many, varied, complex, and lasted several months. Many were destructive, trivializing, discounting, and disdainful of our prior achievements. Most people were immobilized; many students were injured and silenced. Conflict avoidance became normative. Accommodations flourished. Manipulations escalated.

The series of events concluded with my resignation as director. I left the table. To clarify my decision, I shared with faculty and students this book's chapter on leaving the table. Every word there fit, and helped me make this decision and act upon it. I was a bit bemused that I actually had a chapter in a book to share with others in an attempt to explain my decision. I was also startled at how well it fit. I was living at a new depth the lessons of the book.

I went in search of a new table and a new dialogue. During this lengthy process, however, I found the depth of meaning I had been searching for. Looking back, I knew I thought of this program as the best expression in my career of my leadership and professional creativity as a nurse educator. Harms to the program and to me went deeper, losses were more painful. Looking at the past as prologue, I concluded that this must be the upper-division course. I learned a lot.

Useful Addenda

Here are some additional things I learned about negotiating at an uneven table.

When a person has a high need for control, a person refusing to be controlled by that person can be perceived as engaging in controlling behavior. Hence, if I elect to exercise moral agency, and another needs to control me, I may actually appear controlling because I thwart the goal of the other. This may be a simple case of projection of the shadow, but it feels a bit more complex than that to me. Helping people see that refusing to be controlled is not controlling behavior has proven to be a sizable challenge. It is a complex task, at best.

Projection of one's shadow can be an occasional flaw, or a defensive behavior. I had never realized it could be a lifestyle. When a person uses this dynamic as a lifestyle, it taints everything. If that person has influence in an organization, it can even taint the whole organization. It takes a great deal of courage to confront a person who is projecting his or her shadow on you. It is actually a fairly impressive example of Gandhi's description of creating the conditions for interpersonal violence and risking it. Retaliation can be very seductive under these conditions. Retaliation can also be dishonestly explained as self-defense. Discrimination becomes imperative. So does truth telling.

The Louis L'Amour system of managing violence (see Chapter Six) is itself a moral system, where the end justifies the means. I was raised in the Midwest, where the end never justifies the means. If nothing else, a midwesterner would view this as impractical. I sometimes think it is based on our relationship with the land. You can abuse the land to get a crop, but you will always pay for it.

I have never been able to complete a L'Amour book, a fact that amuses all my brothers. I can hear his justifiable violence lurking. In some parts of the United States, among some groups, for some individuals, the L'Amour moral code prevails. The end justifies the means when dominant power is part of a process, and one of the acceptable means can be interpersonal violence. This code can shape everything that happens at the table. I'm not certain, but it may be a table one should never go to, or when discovered, leave immediately.

The most central factor that identifies a behavior as manipulative is the intent to deceive. In a moral system where the end justifies the means, the desire to seek a perceived good can lead to manipulations that may be defended as justifiable violence. Deception, under these conditions, can appear to be virtuous. The virtue, it is argued, is the intent of the end, the goal sought. One does what one must do to get this fine goal. Lying really is OK because I really do mean well.

When this is a cultural norm, it shapes all negotiations and is the assumption at every table. It is a particularly virulent version of unevenness, since it involves moral disadvantage. If I hold myself to a moral code where the end does not justify the means, then claimers prevail simply because their ends have no moral anchor. They may also find considerable cultural support because their rationale of ends justifying means is normative, perhaps even viewed as intelligent and virtuous. If one leaves a table where this is the norm, the need of claimers to "win" may escalate simply as an expression of defending this cultural norm.

Multiple worldviews residing together is a difficult challenge if any given player needs to have the best or right worldview. I find a distinction made by Walter Truett Anderson (1995) useful in this regard. One need not embrace the philosophical systems that posit or describe postmodernism. One does not, however, have the option of ignoring postmodernity, the state we are in.

We are slogging our way toward adaptation to a postmodern world with grave discomforts. Perhaps the greatest discomfort is discovering our need to be right, to prevail: the sense of entitlement of the claimer. To prevail, discrediting the others can become the primary focus of discourse. Difference and diversity are very real threats for claimers.

This is a sophisticated intellectualized version of claiming behavior. It is also increasingly a stance taken by persons who believed that they were entitled, and see that entitlement eroding. We may give lip service to multiculturalism. It is no longer, however, a discussion about minorities. It is a discussion about majorities in most cities. Those who most cherished the dominant paradigm continue to run just about everything, but their numbers are declining, their hegemony is deteriorating, and they are not particularly graceful in the evolutionary moment. The death throes of the patriarchy are not attractive to watch.

Health care has as its primary premise to "do no harm." This easily focuses on patients and their families. It is less clear if it applies to all the persons one encounters in the health care community. Indeed, doing harm to others in order to do no harm to the patients is sometimes defended. Moral confusion exacerbates this situation.

Integrity and wholeness are sometimes viewed as synonymous. Wholeness in this sense refers to all aspects of being human. The word integrity is commonly used to refer to moral integrity. Wholeness, however, would posit that all dimensions of what it means to be a human seek integrity: physical, emotional, intellectual, moral, social, and spiritual. To neglect one is to neglect others. Intellectual integrity and moral integrity are closely linked. It is difficult to exercise moral integrity if intellectual integrity is compromised, and vice versa. This is a subtle insight. Moral or intellectual confusion or laziness can exacerbate the challenge.

A materialistic culture develops a conceptualization of violence that is physical in nature. Interpersonal violence, violence against a spirit or soul, emotional violence, social violence, moral violence; these manifestations are more difficult to recognize as violent, more readily viewed as simple expressions of human nature. A robust understanding of nonviolence would include all the dimensions of being human. These are all the ways we can be violent to one another. And these are all the ways we need to heal.

Manipulation can be covert enough that it is only evident in retrospect. These situations demonstrate the need for great care in expanding the context. The context may include persons who elect to not be at the table in order to engage in covert manipulations not apparent at the table. Under such conditions, the table can become farcical because the actual negotiations are manipulations conducted elsewhere. Claimers who need to prevail may view this as a preferred approach to conflict. Leaving the table will not significantly alter this dynamic, and finding new tables becomes the wisest course of action.

People in leadership roles have unique responsibilities in relationship to conflict and its resolution. Failure to address this compromises their effectiveness as leaders, and the effectiveness of their organizations. Conflict avoidance is not peacekeeping, and can actually be a fairly cruel and violent behavior. Conflict accommodation can draw an entire organization into compromised integrity. Leaders count.

Conflict avoidance can be fear masquerading as kindness, goodness of spirit, even nobility. It can also trigger denial of the shadow, followed closely by projection. It is difficult to discriminate when someone is projecting his or her shadow on you. I have to own my own dark side carefully and honestly before I can ascertain the degree to which people may be projecting their shadow on me. Once that discernment process is completed, it is important to not take in the other person's shadow, but return it to them. It is theirs to own. They may neither understand this nor thank you, but it is important to refuse to take in another's dark side. It has been my experience that I have enough of my own without taking in wandering chunks of someone else's. This takes a lot of time and energy, but it is worth it.

Structured deliberate efforts to create something that images our preferred future can be dangerous, and the "thing" itself can be a very vulnerable creature. This new thing deliberately challenges the status quo simply by its existence. Although liberation and creativity can be wonderful, and though the imagined possible can be an extraordinary adventure, such creatures are also places where reestablishing the uneven table becomes a top priority for those attached to the past. Galileo's story is an important lesson.

So too with Mohandas Gandhi and Martin Luther King Jr., the key proponents and avatars of interpersonal nonviolence. Not only can people get very grumpy when you attempt to find constructive ways to be at uneven tables; sometimes they can get homicidal. These are consequences one may have taken on and it is useful to recognize this fact. I ponder that these two heroes, two persons who shaped my thinking, were both assassinated. I am not sure why I didn't notice that before. I think I didn't want to do so. Fear counts.

In any failed negotiation, both parties bear some responsibility for failure. The words that fit this situation are the words "I am sorry." This is not so much an admission of guilt but an acknowledgement of responsibility. If it is viewed as an admission of guilt, there is little to be done about this. Taking responsibility for one's own failures continues to be a moral choice worth embracing.

The good done never disappears. It lurks in the hearts of those who grew and were enriched by that good. Tables change. Dialogues change. Good persists. It is important to remember this when leaving a table.

If my behavior evokes interpersonal violence and I elect not to retaliate, this can escalate the violence. The rage that triggered the violence is counting on retaliation, ready for it, prepared. Its absence can be enraging. This doubles the risk of truth telling and drawing your line in the sand without cruelty.

Your lens can always get larger.

Claimers always win a conflict when seated at a table with creators. It is increasingly unclear why this fixation could be perceived as a good thing. To have claimed successfully and in the process silenced and harmed others is destructive of life energy. If I harm others, I harm myself. I can always achieve more from creative synergy than from even the most stunning performance as a claimer. Claiming is even dumber than I thought.

It is hard to be good at this work. Others may like the ideas, but view the moral challenge as excessive. It is important to notice this.

Pride actually does go before the fall.

Every fall is a new beginning, a humiliation that takes us back to our humanity, and opens new pathways of learning and loving. When what is now falls apart, the space is created for something new.

Humor really helps.

Skill Building

All of these new lessons have served as a catalyst for me, an impetus to continue my work, and expand it. As is perhaps apparent, it was not easy for me to write this progress report. Truth telling can be costly. Nonetheless, these experiences have not only intensified my commitment to the work of creative negotiation. It has also motivated me to write the next book beyond this one, one where I hope to further explain the skills needed and often undeveloped in people not born to the table.

I am struck by the hunger many people express who hope to become more constructive about their responses to conflict. I am humbled by the courage of people to keep trying to master those skills, knowing full well their cost. I am particularly touched by the persons I have taught who, despite deep and old habits of conflict avoidance, are trying to find new approaches to this challenge. These persons have become for me a community of support and hope.

I am also sobered by the growing evidence of the cost and uselessness of our culture's fixation on dominance power, and the intensity with which those who believed themselves entitled struggle with cultural changes over which they have little or no control. My daughters and their peers give me hope, because they seem less enamored than their elders with this fixation on entitlement and dominant power. Perhaps an era is passing and we are called upon to wish it speed and give it a good funeral.

Edging toward sixty, I ponder the life lessons that make me ready to not only continue this work, but to do so with greater wisdom and patience. I am with Norman Cousins on this one: I really do think there is a better world waiting to be created, and I want to be on the creative team. When I made my decision to leave the table of our doctoral program, I wrote a poem about that turning point. It seems a good way to end this chapter.

Athena

Athena retires: in repose on the
Green glider, in late noon shadow
On the side porch, soft as sand, gritty;
She is watching the drama unfurling
In the front yard, she is calculating odds.

Athena observes: vigilant and reflective,
Is was never her job to keep others alive,
Rather to model full life living despite
Unsupportable odds: nothing stronger
In sight, nothing likely to show up.

Athena rises at midnight, silent to the
Back kitchen, nodding and noting, she
Gives advice and counsel, she smiles then,
And recollects the history and the now, and
Points out endless possibilities and laughs.

Athena perdures, and calls a halt to all war,
Sculpts imaginings and new dancings and
Stands still as stone in the hurricane times:
She can explain herself to anyone and has
Decided to explain herself to no one.

—pbk

29

Imagining the Future
An Invitation to Continue the Dance

You may recall that at the beginning of this book I told you I wanted this to start a conversation. I am drawing to the close of my part of initiating this conversation. You, I assume, are now aware of some of your reactions to the book. My final comments are about those reactions.

If you liked this book, I would really enjoy hearing from you about what you liked and why you liked it. This helps me know more, improve my capacity to innovate, and most important, helps us both stay in the dialogue. Between the first and second editions of this book, a large number of people did just that. It is a pleasure to take the time right now to thank you. Every observation proved useful, many invaluable.

If you liked this book but also have a hunch that in reading it you found some of my distortions, misconceptions, or limitations, I'd like to hear from you too. I may simply agree with you, but that too is part of a dialogue. If you want to tell me that my window on reality is partial, all I can really say is that I warned you about that in the beginning. I never thought this was the whole of reality, and I have tried to assure you of that throughout the book. Everything I wrote here was uniquely through my lens on reality. The fact that it is not the same as yours was something I acknowledged at the outset, and reaffirm. That is why there is a dialogue, to share these lenses so we can all grow, learn, and expand our worldviews. Some of you have done exactly this, and I have learned a great deal from these lens-enlarging exchanges. I thank you for your generous gifts.

You may therefore have insights that my comments triggered that you suspect I may not know about and need to be told. I would really like to know about this. Check it out first though, and make sure that you are not repackaging some old reality; after fifty-eight years, having people selling me old repackaged realities does not capture my interest much. You may also be stimulated to imagine well beyond my limits. That would please me. If you get others to do the same, that would please me even more. What would please me the most is if you have a lot of fun doing this. Some of you, particularly my many students, have done just that, and the pleasure was even greater than I had imagined. These experiences have given me the opportunity for yet more gratitude.

Finally, I need to speak directly to those of you who really don't like what I have to say in this book and really want to tell me about it in no uncertain terms. If it makes you angry, I can feel some degree of compassion for you, but I'm not really interested in just hearing you be angry. I've been at uneven tables for a long time now, and anger gets pretty boring. If you must express your anger, buy a second copy of the book and destroy it ritually. This will do less harm, and of course I can anticipate a small profit from this act. Then reflect on the book for six months. Then, if you still think I need to be saved from the error of my ways, let me know. This too is a dialogue. It probably warrants mentioning that I did get one really angry letter and a few tepid or tedious ones. I learned from these also, sometimes tracking into whole new vistas of insight. I am grateful for these opportunities.

It is my hope that for every person that reads this book, some new approach to dealing with an uneven table will in time emerge and make us all a bit more hopeful about dealing with conflict. It is also my hope that it will create many new dialogues and that they will be ones we will all want to stay in for a very long time.

Finally, I want to end this conversation with a note of encouragement, a summing up of the reasons that moved me to write here what I have written. As this book progressed, I progressed with it, facing new struggles and challenges, discovering new deterrents to my own evolution, facing new faces of fear and limitation and celebrating new faces of honesty and courage.

Why bother with conflict resolution, anyway? Well, because conflict is central to the human condition. As I noted earlier, all conflict is inevitably inner conflict mirroring itself outward to our external world. To have faced the conflicts "out there" more constructively is to have faced the conflicts within more constructively. We are ultimately a social species, and while we can live hermetic lives, they are ones lacking in passion, joy, pleasure, and fulfillment. To reach out to others is to risk conflict, indeed to ensure it, since all human interaction carries that risk and opportunity. In my day-to-day living with others, I manifest my inner uncertainties, confusion, and errors, and these are the stuff of the conflicts I experience.

Thus, if I want a more whole and fulfilled life, if I want to struggle toward my own evolution and enhance the evolution of others, I will risk conflict. Because we are all fractured and limited creatures, we will inevitably experience most conflicts as ones where we in part feel unequal to others and to the task. Tools to deal with the sense of being unequal are thus tools for fuller living, for evolving, and ultimately for loving well.

Whenever I find myself struggling with this challenge and uncertain about which path to take, I find that writing my own epitaph clarifies things. What do I want the summary statement of my life on this planet to be? How will it read? What do I hope is said of me? Some statements I have a clear grasp of, some are still evolving, some I have not yet imagined. Over time, I have found this exercise useful in clarifying my choices. This is not a destination so much as a process, a life process.

Examples may help. I know, for instance, that I want my epitaph to say these things: she was invited to cynicism daily, and she said no; she did not shrink from the challenge of living but held life with both hands and lived it with as much energy and consciousness as she could muster; she was born with limited supplies of humility, patience, and courage but faced these deficits and worked hard to discover abundance; when required to choose, she preferred wisdom to knowledge and truth to safety; through her failures and mistakes, she found compassion; she cherished her personal integrity, sometimes at a great cost; she learned to love well.

I have written this book in the spirit of those statements. As a final exercise, I encourage you to write your own epitaph.

Postscript: September 11, 2001

As the work of this book neared completion, planet Earth tilted on its axis through a series of unimagined events, and I tilted with it. It seems that neither the Earth nor I have fully righted ourselves, and that we will be about this task for some time. Failure to note this tilt, however, is not an option.

We seem startled at our own complex tensions, pulled between a shadowy primal rage and a tender compassion for those who have suffered, and will continue to suffer. We found some new depths in both our generosity and our vengeance. When we muster hope, we are not entirely sure what we are hoping for, or why. There is often a focused effort at connection among us, and we seem unable to even note this fact. Our national identity as *warrior* has erupted, often overshadowing both our reason and our compassion as we ponder our status as *victim*.

In the two months following September 11th, I have conducted workshops on the content of this book with six different groups of participants, in South Carolina, California, Massachusetts, Colorado, Maine, and Texas. Regional differences diffuse in the face of this global tilt. It has seemed to me that we are alternately eager to learn better ways to resolve our conflicts, and fretful that we have failed—and will continue to fail—to do so.

I have always thought that the ideas in this book were my small contribution to the work of peacebuilding. Norman Cousins' observation, quoted at the beginning of this book, haunts me now with greater urgency: "Beyond the clamor of clashing ideologies and the preening and jostling of sovereign tribes, a safer and more responsible world is waiting to be created" (Cousins, 1987, p. 208). It is my hope that this book provides some readers with a means to better participate in that creation.

I have no assurance that the book, or my work, will do so. I do know, however, that it creates a space for me in the community of persons working toward constructive responses to conflict, and that during times of great violence, the members of this community perforce are called upon to intensify their efforts as an antidote to that violence. In a world intent on retaliation, fearful to do otherwise and uncertain about alternatives, there is still a need for healers. Indeed there is a greater need for healers.

At the outset I noted that this book was motivated by the children of planet Earth. I am more certain in my silences about September 11, 2001 than I am in my speaking and writing. We are crafting a sobering legacy for these children. I reserve my deepest silences for them, reflecting often on the story we are collectively writing, yet personally writing to pursue an alternative to the one on my TV, and hoping that you, the reader, will join me in the effort.

Recommended Readings

Allport, G. W. *The Nature of Prejudice*. New York: Doubleday, 1958.

Anderson, W. T. (ed.) *The Truth About the Truth: De-Confusing and Re-Constructing the Postmodern World*. New York: Tarcher/Putnam, 1995.

Arbinger Institute. *Leadership and Self-Deception: Getting out of the Box*. San Francisco: Berrett-Koehler, 2000.

Arendt, H. *Eichmann in Jerusalem: A Report on the Banality of Evil*. New York: Penguin, 1963.

Beck, R. *Nonviolent Story: Narrative Conflict Resolution in the Gospel of Mark*. Maryknoll, N.Y.: Orbis, 1996.

Becker, E. *The Denial of Death*. New York: Free Press, 1973.

Belenky, M. F., Clinchy, B., Goldberger, N. R., and Tarule, J. M. *Women's Ways of Knowing*. New York: Basic Books, 1986.

Berger, J., and others. *Ways of Seeing*. New York: Penguin, 1972.

Berke, J. H. *The Tyranny of Malice*. New York: Summit, 1988.

Bohm, D. *Wholeness and the Implicate Order*. Boston: Ark, 1980.

Bohm, D., and Peat, F. D. *Science, Order, and Creativity*. New York: Bantam, 1987.

Bonhoeffer, D. *Letters and Papers from Prison*. (E. Bethge, ed.) New York: Macmillan, 1971.

Buber, M. *I and Thou*. (2nd ed.) New York: Macmillan, 1958.

Capra, F. *The Tao of Physics*. Boulder: Shambhala, 1975.

Capra, F. *The Turning Point: Science, Society, and the Rising Culture*. New York: Free Press, 1982.

Capra, F. *Uncommon Wisdom: Conversations with Remarkable People*. New York: Bantam, 1988.

Carse, J. P. *Finite and Infinite Games: A Vision of Play and Possibility.* New York: Free Press, 1986.

Christ, C. P. *Laughter of Aphrodite.* New York: HarperCollins, 1987.

Cleveland, H. *The Knowledge Executive.* New York: Truman Talley, 1985.

Coelho, P. *The Pilgrimage: A Contemporary Quest for Ancient Wisdom.* San Francisco: HarperSanFrancisco, 1992.

Coles, R. *Lives of Moral Leadership.* New York: Random House, 2000.

Connolly, M. *Mr. Blue.* New York: Doubleday, 1954.

Cousins, N. *The Pathology of Power.* New York: Norton, 1987.

De Pree, M. *Leadership is an Art.* New York: Doubleday, 1989.

Dewey, J. *Individualism: Old and New.* New York: Capricorn, 1929.

Einstein, A. *Essays in Humanism.* New York: Philosophical Library, 1983.

Eisenstein, H. *Contemporary Feminist Thought.* Boston: Hall, 1983.

Eisler, R. *The Chalice and the Blade.* New York: HarperCollins, 1987.

Eliade, M. *The Sacred and the Profane: The Nature of Religion.* Orlando: Harcourt Brace, 1957.

Eliot, T. S. *The Complete Poems and Plays: 1909–1950.* Orlando: Harcourt Brace, 1963.

Emerson, R. W. *Self-Reliance.* White Plains, N.Y.: Peter Pauper, 1967.

Estes, C. P. *Women Who Run with the Wolves.* New York: Ballantine, 1992.

Ferguson, M. *The Aquarian Conspiracy.* Los Angeles: Tarcher, 1980.

Ferguson, M. *PragMagic.* New York: Pocket Books, 1987.

Frankl, V. E. *Man's Search for Meaning.* Boston: Beacon, 1959.

Fromm, E. *To Have or to Be?* New York: Bantam, 1976.

Frost, R. *The Poetry of Robert Frost: The Collected Poems.* (E. C. Lathem, ed.). Austin: Holt, Rinehart and Winston, 1969.

Fuller, R. B. *Intuition.* (2nd ed.) San Luis Obispo, Calif.: Impact, 1983.

Gardner, H. *The Mind's New Science.* New York: Basic Books, 1985.

Gardner, J. W. *Self-Renewal: The Individual and the Innovative Society.* New York: HarperCollins, 1963.

Gardner, J. W. *Excellence: Can We Be Equal and Excellent Too?* (Rev. ed.) New York: Norton, 1984.

Gandhi, M. *An Autobiography: The Story of My Experiments with Truth.* Boston: Beacon, 1993.

Gandhi, M. *Book of Prayers.* Berkeley: Berkeley Hills Books, 1999.

Gilligan, C. *In a Different Voice: Psychological Theory and Women's Development.* Cambridge, Mass.: Harvard University Press, 1982.

Gleick, J. *Chaos: Making a New Science.* New York: Penguin, 1987.

Gould, S. J. *The Mismeasure of Man.* New York: Norton, 1981.

Gruen, A. *The Betrayal of the Self: The Fear of Autonomy in Men and Women.* (H. Hannum and H. Hannum, trans.) New York: Grove, 1988.

Gyatso, T. *Freedom in Exile: The Autobiography of the Dalai Lama.* New York: HarperCollins, 1990.

Gyatso, T. *The Power of Compassion: A Collection of Lectures by His Holiness the XIV Dalai Lama.* London, UK: HarperCollins, 1995.

Gyatso, T. *Ancient Wisdom, Modern World: Ethics for a New Millennium by the Dalai Lama.* London, UK: Little, Brown, 1999.

Hart, P., and Montaldo, J. (eds.) *The Intimate Merton: His Life from His Journals.* New York: HarperCollins, 1999.

Hillman, J. *Kinds of Power: A Guide to Its Intelligent Uses.* New York: Doubleday, 1995.

Hillman, J. *The Force of Character and the Lasting Life.* New York: Random House, 1999.

Hock, D. *Birth of the Chaordic Age.* San Francisco: Berrett-Koehler, 1999.

Hoffer, E. *The True Believer: Thoughts on the Nature of Mass Movements.* New York: HarperCollins, 1951.

Hoffer, E. *The Ordeal of Change.* New York: HarperCollins, 1952.

Houston, J. *The Hero and the Goddess.* New York: Ballantine, 1992.

Howe, N., and Strauss, B. *13th Gen: Abort, Retry, Ignore, Fail?* New York: Vintage, 1993.

Johnson, R. A., and Ruhl, J. M. *Contentment: A Way to True Happiness.* New York: HarperCollins, 1999.

Jones, R. S. *Physics as Metaphor.* New York: Meridian, 1982.

Jung, C. *The Undiscovered Self.* New York: Mentor, 1958.

Jung, C. *Memories, Dreams, Reflections.* (A. Jaffe, ed.) New York: Vintage, 1963.

Koestler, A. *The Roots of Coincidence.* New York: Vintage, 1972.

Koestler, A. *Janus: A Summing up.* New York: Vintage, 1978.

Kopp, S. *An End to Innocence: Facing Life Without Illusions.* Toronto: Bantam, 1978.

Krishnamurti, J., and Bohm, D. *The Future of Humanity.* New York: HarperCollins, 1986.

Kuhn, T. S. *The Structure of Scientific Revolutions.* (2nd ed.) Chicago: University of Chicago Press, 1970.

Lakoff, G., and Johnson, M. *Metaphors We Live by.* Chicago: University of Chicago Press, 1980.

Laudan, L. *Progress and Its Problems: Towards a Theory of Scientific Growth.* Berkeley: University of California Press, 1977.

Maslow, A. H. (ed.). *New Knowledge in Human Values.* South Bend, Ind.: Regnery/Gateway, 1959.

May, R. *The Courage to Create*. New York: Bantam, 1975.

May, R. *The Discovery of Being*. New York: Norton, 1983.

May, R. *My Quest for Beauty*. New York: Saybrook, 1985.

Mayerhoff, M. *On Caring*. New York: Perennial Library, 1971.

Mead, G. H. *On Social Psychology*. Chicago: University of Chicago Press, 1984.

Merton, T. *Thoughts in Solitude*. New York: Farrar, Straus & Giroux, 1956.

Merton, T. *Faith and Violence: Christian Teaching and Christian Practice*. Notre Dame, Ind.: University of Notre Dame Press, 1968.

Merton, T. *Contemplation in a World of Action*. Notre Dame, Ind.: University of Notre Dame Press, 1998.

Miller, J. A. *The Way of Suffering: A Geography of Crisis*. Washington, D.C.: Georgetown University Press, 1988.

Miller, J. B. *Toward a New Psychology of Women*. Boston: Beacon, 1976.

Montagu, A., and Matson, F. *The Dehumanization of Man*. New York: McGraw-Hill, 1983.

Moore, T. *Care of the Soul: A Guide for Cultivating Depth and Sacredness in Everyday Life.* New York: HarperCollins, 1992.

Moses, J. *Oneness: Great Principles Shared by All Religions*. New York: Ballantine, 1989.

Moustakas, C. E. *The Self: Explorations in Personal Growth*. New York: Harper-Collins, 1956.

Nair, K. *A Higher Standard of Leadership: Lessons from the Life of Gandhi*. San Francisco: Berrett-Koehler, 1994.

Neihardt, J. G. *Black Elk Speaks: Being the Life Story of a Holy Man of the Oglala Sioux*. Lincoln: University of Nebraska Press, 1979.

Nietzsche, F. *Beyond Good and Evil*. Chicago: Regnery, 1955.

Peat, F. D. *Synchronicity: The Bridge Between Matter and Mind*. New York: Bantam, 1987.

Percy, W. *The Thanatos Syndrome*. New York: Ivy, 1987.

Pirsig, R. M. *Lila: An Inquiry into Morals*. New York: Bantam, 1991.

Prigogine, I., and Stengers, I. *Order out of Chaos: Man's New Dialogue with Nature*. New York: Bantam, 1984.

Progoff, I. *Jung, Synchronicity, and Human Destiny: C. G. Jung's Theory of Meaningful Coincidence*. New York: Julian Press, 1973.

Progoff, I. *The Dynamics of Hope: Perspectives of Process in Anxiety and Creativity, Imagery and Dreams*. New York: Dialogue House Library, 1985.

Reason, P., and Rowan, J. *Human Inquiry: A Source Book of New Paradigm Research*. New York: Wiley, 1981.

Robbins, T. *Skinny Legs and All*. New York: Bantam, 1990.

Schur, E. M. *Labeling Women Deviant: Gender, Stigma, and Social Control*. New York: Random House, 1984.

Seelig, C. (ed.). *Ideas and Opinions: Albert Einstein*. New York: Crown, 1982.

Solovyov, V. *The Meaning of Love*. (T. R. Beyer, trans., ed.). West Stockbridge, Mass.: Lindisfarne, 1985. (Originally published 1945)

Sontag, S. *Illness as a Metaphor and AIDS and Its Metaphors*. New York: Doubleday, 1990.

Teilhard de Chardin, P. *Hymn of the Universe*. New York: HarperCollins, 1965a.

Teilhard de Chardin, P. *The Phenomenon of Man*. (2nd ed.) New York: HarperCollins, 1965b.

Tillich, P. *The Courage to Be*. New Haven, Conn.: Yale University Press, 1952.

Walker, B. B. *The I Ching or Book of Changes*. New York: St. Martin's Press, 1992.

Welch, S. D. *A Feminist Ethic of Risk*. Minneapolis: Fortress Press, 1990.

Wheatley, M. J. *Leadership and the New Science: Learning About Organization from an Orderly Universe*. San Francisco: Berrett-Koehler, 1992.

Whyte, D. *Crossing the Unknown Sea: Work as a Pilgrimage of Identity*. New York: Riverhead, 2001.

Wilber, K. *No Boundary: Eastern and Western Approaches to Personal Growth*. Boston: Shambhala, 1979.

Wilber, K. (ed.). *Quantum Questions: Mystical Writings of the World's Greatest Physicists*. Boston: Shambhala, 1984.

Zukav, G. *The Dancing Wu-Li Masters: An Overview of the New Physics*. New York: Morrow, 1979.

Zukav, G. *The Seat of the Soul*. New York: Simon & Schuster, 1989.

Zweig, C., and Wolf, S. *Romancing the Shadow: Illuminating the Dark Side of the Soul*. New York: Ballantine, 1997.

References

Aiken, L. H., and Sage, W. M. "Staffing National Health Care Reform: A Role for Advanced Practice Nurses." *Akron Law Review*, 1993, 26(2), 187–211.

Alinsky, S. D. *Rules for Radicals*. New York: Random House, 1971.

Allport, G. W. *The Nature of Prejudice*. New York: Doubleday, 1958.

Anderson, W. T. (ed.) *The Truth About the Truth: De-Confusing and Re-Constructing the Postmodern World*. New York: Tarcher/Putnam, 1995.

Arendt, H. *Eichmann in Jerusalem: A Report on the Banality of Evil*. New York: Penguin, 1963.

Baker Miller, J. *Toward a New Psychology of Women*. Boston: Beacon, 1987.

Beck, R. *Nonviolent Story: Narrative Conflict Resolution in the Gospel of Mark*. Maryknoll, N.Y.: Orbis, 1996.

Bok, S. *Lying: Moral Choice in Public and Private Life*. New York: Random House, 1978.

Carse, J. P. *Finite and Infinite Games: A Vision of Play and Possibility*. New York: Free Press, 1986.

Cousins, N. *The Pathology of Power*. New York: Norton, 1987.

Eliot, T. S. *Burnt Norton*. In *Four Quartets*. Orlando: Harcourt Brace, 1943.

Farrell, W. *The Myth of Male Power*. New York: Simon & Schuster, 1993.

Freire, P. *Pedagogy of the Oppressed*. New York: Continuum, 1997.

French, J.R.P., and Raven, B. H. "The Bases of Power." In E. P. Hollander and R. G. Hunt (eds.), *Current Perspectives in Social Psychology*. New York: Oxford University Press, 1963.

Frost, R. *The Poetry of Robert Frost: The Collected Poems*. (E. C. Lathem, ed.). Austin: Holt, Rinehart and Winston, 1969.

Harman, W. W. "A Re-Examination of the Metaphysical Foundations of Modern Science." (Causality Issues in Contemporary Science, Research Report CP-1). Sausalito, Calif.: Institute of Noetic Sciences, 1991.

Hillman, J. *Kinds of Power: A Guide to Its Intelligent Uses*. New York: Doubleday, 1995.

Johnson, R. A., and Ruhl, J. M. *Contentment: A Way to True Happiness*. New York: HarperCollins, 1999.

Jung, C. *The Undiscovered Self*. New York: Mentor, 1958.

Jung, C. *Memories, Dreams, Reflections*. (A. Jaffe, ed.). New York: Vintage, 1963.

Koestler, A. *Janus: A Summing up*. New York: Vintage, 1978.

Kritek, P. B. (ed.). *Reflections on Healing: A Central Nursing Construct*. New York: National League for Nursing Press, 1997.

Kuhn, T. S. *The Structure of Scientific Revolutions*. (2nd ed.) Chicago: University of Chicago Press, 1970.

Lakoff, G., and Johnson, M. *Metaphors We Live by*. Chicago: University of Chicago Press, 1980.

Mead, G. H. *On Social Psychology*. Chicago: University of Chicago Press, 1984.

Merton, T. (ed.). *Gandhi on Non-Violence: Selected Texts from Mohandas K. Gandhi's Non-Violence in Peace and War*. Boston: Shambhala, 1996.

Mitchell, E. "Frontier Developments in Consciousness Studies Produce New Medical Advances." Paper presented at the Institute of Noetic Sciences Seventh Annual Conference, Kansas City, Mo., July 1998.

Pirsig, R. M. *Lila: An Inquiry into Morals*. New York: Bantam, 1991.

Raiffa, H. *The Art and Science of Negotiation*. Cambridge, Mass.: Harvard University Press, 1982.

Robbins, T. *Skinny Legs and All*. New York: Bantam, 1990.

Walker, B. B. *The I Ching or Book of Changes*. New York: St. Martin's Press, 1992.

Zweig, C., and Wolf, S. *Romancing the Shadow: Illuminating the Dark Side of the Soul*. New York: Ballantine, 1997.

Index